MORE
DEVOTIONS FOR

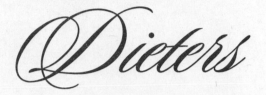

SELECTIONS FROM THE
BEST-SELLING DAILY DEVOTIONAL

DAN R. DICK

BARBOUR
PUBLISHING

MORE
DEVOTIONS FOR

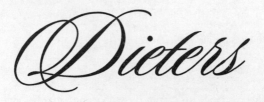

Dieters

ISBN 1-58660-037-0

Published by Barbour Publishing, Inc., P.O. Box 719, Uhrichsville, OH 44683, www.barbourbooks.com

Our mission is to publish and distribute inspirational products offering exceptional value and biblical encouragement to the masses.

Member of the
Evangelical Christian
Publishers Association

Printed in the United States of America.
5 4 3 2 1

DAY 1

Let us therefore come boldly unto the throne of grace, that we may obtain mercy, and find grace to help in time of need. HEBREWS 4:16

Jeffrey never wanted to put anybody out. Instead of asking for help, he would struggle along on his own. Often, Jeffrey didn't get anything accomplished because he refused to impose on anyone else.

Sometimes, we act that way with God. We ask ourselves why God would be interested in helping us solve our problems. The thing is, God wants us to come to Him with our heartfelt needs. We have been invited to come before the throne of grace, and that includes with our diets. When we're honest, we'll admit that we need help, and there is no greater source of help than God.

TODAY'S THOUGHT: Our hope to lose weight becomes reality when we put our trust in God.

DAY 2

I count all things but loss for the excellency of the knowledge of Christ Jesus my Lord: for whom I have suffered the loss of all things, and do count them but dung, that I may win Christ. PHILIPPIANS 3:8

A young man dreamed that he was standing before a table spread with a wide array of tantalizing foods. Beyond the table stood Jesus. The young man began eating the food, and he became completely engrossed in his consumption. When he finished, Jesus was gone, and he didn't know where to look to find Him.

Whenever we engage in gluttony of any kind, our attention is turned from Christ to our own selfish wants. There should be nothing more important in our lives than doing what is pleasing to God. He wants us to be the best we can possibly be. Food, and our love of food, should always take a second place to our love of the Lord.

TODAY'S THOUGHT: Eating pleases me; dieting pleases God!

DAY 3

And let us not be weary in well doing: for in due season we shall reap,
if we faint not.   GALATIANS 6:9

Gwen hadn't seen Ed in almost five years. When they had last been together, she had been very overweight. She had struggled and fought to lose over the years, and she was quite proud of what she had accomplished. She could hardly wait to see his reaction. That was one of the best things about losing weight: seeing the faces of old friends who could hardly recognize you. The looks she got made the fight worthwhile. Their disbelief made Gwen feel she had performed a miracle. Good things truly did come to those who waited and stuck to their hope. God had blessed her a hundredfold.

TODAY'S THOUGHT: What I lose today in weight will be gain in other ways tomorrow!

DAY 4

When wisdom entereth into thine heart, and knowledge is pleasant unto
thy soul; discretion shall preserve thee, understanding shall keep thee:
That thou mayest walk in the way of good men, and keep the paths of
the righteous.   PROVERBS 2:10–11, 20

Knowing what is right and doing what is right are completely different matters. Jessica knew she should lose weight, and she knew the way to do that was to cut back on what she was eating. The problem was that she didn't want to give up any of the foods she loved. She just wasn't committed enough. A friend of hers told her that she had all the knowledge she needed in her head, but none of it was in her heart. The reason she couldn't stick to her diet was that she didn't want to lose weight badly enough. When we find ourselves lacking the proper desire, we need to turn to the Lord to ask His strength for doing what we know to be right.

TODAY'S THOUGHT: Dieting is more than a matter of the mind. It's a matter of the heart!

DAY 5

In your patience possess ye your souls.   LUKE 21:19

Arlene asked the Lord for just a little more patience. She looked at the clock. She had eaten lunch just three hours before, and now her stomach was telling her to eat again. She knew she really couldn't need food again so soon. She concentrated all her attention on the project she was working on and repeated again and again that she wasn't hungry. Before she knew it, she was finishing the project, her hunger had died down, and it was almost five o'clock. Quickly, Arlene thanked God for helping her hang on awhile. It wasn't nearly as hard to get by with God giving her strength and support.

TODAY'S THOUGHT: Decide to control your stomach instead of letting it control you!

DAY 6

And ye shall be hated of all men for my name's sake: but he that endureth to the end shall be saved.   MATTHEW 10:22

Christ has a powerful lesson for those who choose to diet. Dieting makes us different, and it is never easy to be different. Being Christians made the disciples different, and they had to suffer many things for their difference. People who are different are often excluded by others. Sometimes they are even abused and persecuted for their differences. There was only one reason the disciples were able to persevere in their faith, and that was the presence of the Holy Spirit in their lives. That same Spirit can give us the power to be different and the strength to persevere, even through a tough diet.

TODAY'S THOUGHT: Jesus Christ helps everyone who chooses to be different!

Day 7

Blessed is the man that endureth temptation: for when he is tried, he shall receive the crown of life, which the Lord hath promised to them that love him.

JAMES 1:12

Christ allows us to declare a special kind of independence from the prison of obesity. Prisoners endure their captivity because they believe that they will one day find release. Through perseverance we earn the right to declare our independence from fat. God will stand with us as we fight for a healthier, more slender body. His Holy Spirit will help us withstand the temptations of rich, fattening foods, and He promises to bless our efforts to do what is right and good. Let us celebrate the freedom from flesh that God will help us achieve.

TODAY'S THOUGHT: Faith in Christ can lead to freedom from fat!

Day 8

We glory in tribulations also: knowing that tribulation worketh patience; and patience, experience; and experience, hope.

ROMANS 5:3–4

The first week had been the toughest. Perry had paced back and forth past the refrigerator a thousand times. His hunger was so intense that it made him feel ill. He stuck with it a week, but he didn't lose much weight. He decided that he would diet at least one more week. Then it happened! A few pounds came off. Perry felt better. He felt more hopeful. The longer he dieted, the easier it got; especially when he could see some results.

Dieting is tough. It takes a lot of patience to wait for the first few results, but when they finally come, they offer us the hope we need to stick with it.

TODAY'S THOUGHT: God gives us hope in order to cope!

Day 9

And let us not be weary in well doing: for in due season we shall reap, if we faint not.   GALATIANS 6:9

Janet was tired of dieting. She had been at it for almost six months. She looked better and knew that she was doing the right thing. Taking the pounds off had been hard, but sometimes Janet felt that keeping them off was even harder. Thin people didn't understand that dieting wasn't just something to do to lose weight. For a person with weight problems, it had to be a way of life.

God knows that dieting is hard. He knows dieting can be a bore. More than that, He knows we need help to diet. Rely on God. He won't let you down.

TODAY'S THOUGHT: I will take dieting one day at a time, one pound at a time!

Day 10

But without faith it is impossible to please him: for he that cometh to God must believe that he is, and that he is a rewarder of them that diligently seek him.   HEBREWS 11:6

Tim always said that God really didn't help him much. The trouble was, Tim never did much for God, either. He rarely prayed, hardly went to church, and didn't even own a Bible. When someone suggested that Tim might go on a diet, he said dieting didn't do any good. Tim pursued a diet about as apathetically as he pursued God.

We will never succeed in anything unless we dedicate ourselves— body, mind, and soul—to achieving our goal. A deep and driving faith can be the perfect model for our diets. If we will strive to lose weight as much as we strive after God, He will bless our effort.

TODAY'S THOUGHT: I'm giving everything I've got to losing weight!

DAY 11

Behold, we count them happy which endure. Ye have heard of the patience of Job, and have seen the end of the Lord; that the Lord is very pitiful, and of tender mercy.   JAMES 5:11

Gretchen wanted the job so badly. The doctor had told her she had to lose twenty pounds in order to pass the physical. Tina and Ann also had to lose weight to join the company. After a couple of weeks, Tina gave up. One week later, Ann folded, too. They both told Gretchen she was wasting her time. Gretchen didn't care. She held on, got her position, and never once regretted all she had to do to get it. She thanked the Lord that she had the strength to hold on when her friends had given up. Without His help, she never would have made it.

TODAY'S THOUGHT: Job lost everything, and God blessed him greatly for what he suffered. If Job can endure, so can I!

DAY 12

Wherefore the rather, brethren, give diligence to make your calling and election sure: for if ye do these things, ye shall never fall.
                    2 PETER 1:10

Beverly never let her Bible get very far away from her. At the first tiny pang of hunger, she grabbed it and immersed herself in the Gospels. Feeding on the Word of God was much better for her than feeding her face, and it always took her mind off her hunger. God wouldn't let her fail. He gave her strength and commitment when she needed it the most. Her diet had helped make her a much stronger person spiritually. She had seen God's power to help her lose weight, and it had given her even more confidence in His power to do other things. Beverly knew that her diligence and perseverance came from God and nowhere else.

TODAY'S THOUGHT: I am keeping God between me and the refrigerator!

Day 13

For I reckon that the sufferings of this present time are not worthy to be compared with the glory which shall be revealed in us.

ROMANS 8:18

Jimmy was fascinated by the cocoon. He watched the caterpillar work on its new home for hours. Every day he came in to look at the cocoon. When the monarch butterfly finally emerged, Jimmy was delighted.

God works some amazing miracles in nature. It shouldn't be so hard to believe that He will work such miracles in the lives of His people. Losing weight might not seem like a miracle, but for those who struggle with their weight, it often feels as if only a miracle will suffice. If God can transform a caterpillar into a beautiful butterfly, He certainly can help us when all we want is to lose weight.

TODAY'S THOUGHT: I am one of God's miracles, and He will help me be my best!

Day 14

But as God hath distributed to every man, as the Lord hath called every one, so let him walk. 1 CORINTHIANS 7:17

Karen got so angry. Her friend Angie had started her diet at the same time Karen had begun. They had shopped together, eaten together, exercised together, but Angie had lost seven pounds more. It wasn't fair. What was the use of dieting when she couldn't lose weight as fast as her friend? She put forth the same effort but got less reward.

God has made each of His children differently. No two are exactly alike. We are called by God to do our best with what we are given. We may not have the same results on our diet that others have on theirs, but that's okay. God will bless us for what we do, and that's what really counts.

TODAY'S THOUGHT: God will help me lose my weight without losing my mind!

DAY 15

For do I now persuade men, or God? or do I seek to please men? for if I yet pleased men, I should not be the servant of Christ.

GALATIANS 1:10

Granny wanted Ellen to lose weight. She used to offer her bribes all the time to encourage her. The problem was, no matter how much weight Ellen lost, her grandmother wanted her to lose more. There was just no pleasing her. Instead of helping Ellen lose weight, Granny just made her more frustrated and discouraged. It wasn't until Ellen decided she wanted to lose weight for herself that it really worked for her. She prayed for God's help, and He delivered. Doing it for Granny wasn't enough; doing it for God and herself made it all worthwhile.

TODAY'S THOUGHT: The more I care, the less I weigh!

DAY 16

For we are his workmanship, created in Christ Jesus unto good works, which God hath before ordained that we should walk in them.

EPHESIANS 2:10

Randy couldn't believe how tough Bob's dad was on Bob. What was even more amazing was that Bob didn't seem to mind. Randy would have gone crazy if his own father had demanded so much from him. Bob told him that his father was really a wonderful person and that he only wanted him to be the best person he could possibly be. Randy found it hard to believe, but one thing he did know: He sure wished he had as close a relationship with his own father as Bob had with his.

Our heavenly Father expects a lot from us. He wants us to be everything we can be. Though He's tough on us at times, He will always stand beside us to help us when we try to improve.

TODAY'S THOUGHT: When we aren't tough enough on ourselves, God will be as tough as we need Him to be!

Day 17

Being confident of this very thing, that he which hath begun a good work in you will perform it until the day of Jesus Christ.

PHILIPPIANS 1:6

Ron was one of the best contractors in the business. Every job he'd ever started, he'd completed to the client's satisfaction. He never left anything undone. His reputation was beyond reproach. No one ever had to worry when they had Ron working for them.

When we rely on God to help us with our dieting, we can rest assured that He will stick with us throughout the entire process. God does not give up. When He begins a job, He finishes it. We can have complete confidence in God. He will help us realize our goal.

TODAY'S THOUGHT: With God's help, I can see this thing through to the end!

Day 18

Whereunto I also labour, striving according to his working, which worketh in me mightily.

COLOSSIANS 1:29

Gail couldn't believe how much her life was changing. All through college, Gail hadn't even set foot in a church. The only social situation she had been comfortable in was where food was involved. College had been lonely and unfulfilling, not to mention fattening. Just recently she had attended church with her new neighbor, and it was like coming home. She felt comfortable and accepted. Her newfound relationship with Jesus Christ gave her a different perspective on her life. She suddenly found a deep concern for her appearance and health. As God became more and more a part of her life, Gail vowed to become the best person she could possibly be.

TODAY'S THOUGHT: God's might is greater than my appetite!

DAY 19

For verily, when we were with you, we told you before that we should suffer tribulation; even as it came to pass, and ye know.

1 THESSALONIANS 3:4

Why don't diets get any easier? Chocolate cake is just as tempting a month or two after you start dieting as it is the day after you start. Time doesn't heal the cravings that go along with diets. There is suffering in dieting. For that reason, a good attitude and strong state of mind are essential for a productive, long-lasting diet. God gives us strength of character and determination. There is no tribulation, even dieting, that God can't get us through. Diets may not ever get easy, but they do get manageable when we add God's strength and perseverance to our own.

TODAY'S THOUGHT: What seems impossible, God makes possible!

DAY 20

And if a man also strive for masteries, yet is he not crowned, except he strive lawfully.   2 TIMOTHY 2:5

Susan lay looking up at the ceiling in her hospital room. She couldn't believe everything had turned out as it had. Jill had promised the pills were safe and that she would lose weight fast. All the pills had done were to make her violently ill and land her in the hospital.

Shortcuts are not the answers. God has given us willpower and miraculous bodies that repair themselves if we give them the chance. Dieting doesn't require chemicals or radical exercising. Dieting requires mastery over our base desires and our selfish natures. Rely on God. We need nothing else.

TODAY'S THOUGHT: God can do more to help me than anything else I could find!

DAY 21

If others be partakers of this power over you, are not we rather? Nevertheless we have not used this power; but suffer all things, lest we should hinder the gospel of Christ.   1 CORINTHIANS 9:12

Betty got so annoyed with Sarah. Sarah had lost so much weight, but whenever anyone asked her how she did it, she told them she couldn't have done it without God's help. That got old really fast. Why didn't she just take credit and let it go at that? Everything had to be a big spiritual production for Sarah!

It's hard for some people to actually realize the power that Christians find in Jesus Christ. They can't understand our gratitude and thankfulness. We are partakers in a great and wonderful power, and it is right for us to acknowledge the source of that power. Christ saves lives, and He liberates us from things like obesity that threaten to make life less than it was meant to be.

TODAY'S THOUGHT: I will give thanks to God for His help in my diet!

DAY 22

I have fought a good fight, I have finished my course, I have kept the faith.   2 TIMOTHY 4:7

Bonnie took a good look in the mirror. Amazing. She never thought she'd look this good again in her life. All the pain, torture, and sacrifice was well worth it. She still couldn't believe it. She had dreamed of the day she would feel really good about her dieting, and that day had arrived. What a great feeling!

If we will persevere, the day of triumph will indeed come. Like Paul, we need to fight the good fight, keep the faith, and complete the course. God promises to reward those who remain steadfast. Hold on to your dream, and God will bless you richly.

TODAY'S THOUGHT: I am closer to my goal with each passing day!

DAY 23

I press toward the mark for the prize of the high calling of God in Christ Jesus. PHILIPPIANS 3:14

Stan lived to please people. He served his church, his job, and his family with total devotion. He was continually asking what he could do for others. There was nothing Stan would not do in order to please someone else. Stan had never worried about his weight until one Sunday when the pastor read that his body was the Lord's temple. From that day forward, Stan worked to make it a fit and healthy temple. Not only was God pleased at Stan's desire to improve himself, but He was also pleased by the example Stan set for others.

TODAY'S THOUGHT: I can actually glorify God just by losing weight!

DAY 24

Continue in prayer, and watch in the same with thanksgiving. COLOSSIANS 4:2

Jane couldn't believe how much harder it was to diet now that Dottie had moved away. The strength and support of having someone to diet with had been immense. Just having someone to talk to had helped a lot. Now there was no one close by to say, "No!" The only thing that was saving Jane was her reliance on God. Whenever she found herself tempted and wishing for Dottie's support, she closed her eyes and talked to God. His presence assured Jane, and she was able to withstand temptation. It was good to have God as close as a prayer. For that she was eternally grateful.

TODAY'S THOUGHT: Help in time of temptation is just one prayer away!

Day 25

Have we not power to eat and to drink?   1 CORINTHIANS 9:4

Kevin blamed the diets. Kevin blamed his friends. Kevin blamed a bad childhood, glands, communists, and a government plot. Kevin blamed everyone but Kevin. Kevin tried, and Kevin failed, but he never learned to take responsibility for his obesity.

We can never hope to get anywhere unless we are willing to take ownership of our own problems. God has given us freedom of choice. We have the ability to abuse that privilege if we so desire. It is our choice, however, and we control our own destiny. Dieting is nothing more than learning to tame a freedom that has degenerated into gluttony. God will help us tame that beast.

TODAY'S THOUGHT: God's in control of my life; my stomach isn't.

Day 26

We ourselves glory in you in the churches of God for your patience and faith in all your persecutions and tribulations that ye endure.
                                                    2 THESSALONIANS 1:4

Ed was on a severely restricted diet by order of his doctor. There were more foods he couldn't have than there were that he could. Almost everyone felt sorry for him, because they knew how much Ed loved his food. The only person who didn't seem to feel sorry for Ed was Ed. He accepted his fate with a smile and a shrug. His ability to adjust was a testimony to his faith and character. Many people found comfort in Ed's ability to take his diet in stride. His perseverance showed many people that it could be done. Through something so simple, God managed to touch the lives of many.

TODAY'S THOUGHT: My diet is only as big a deal as I make it!

Day 27

I will instruct thee and teach thee in the way which thou shalt go: I will guide thee with mine eye. PSALM 32:8

Terry had been a savior. It was so nice to find someone who had gone through a long, hard diet before. God had really brought them together. At the time Lisa needed someone most, Terry had miraculously showed up. Lisa wondered if Terry were an angel in disguise. She had been such a great help.

God often answers our prayers through the people He sends into our lives at key times. It is good to seek out the support of others who can relate to what we're going through. Pray that God will lead you to such people, so they might accompany you through the tough times.

TODAY'S THOUGHT: Help me remember that I'm not alone!

Day 28

This I say then, Walk in the Spirit, and ye shall not fulfil the lust of the flesh. GALATIANS 5:16

Dan made a resolution to use his breakfast and lunch times for prayer and reflection. He would eat something light, then spend the rest of the time in quiet time with God. It got him through some really tough periods of hunger and temptation. Refreshed by the time with God, Dan then no longer felt the desire to stuff himself. God strengthened him, gave him courage, and filled him with resistance enough to persevere.

God will fill the emptiness we feel in our bellies. He will fill us with His own Holy Spirit and lead us away from temptation. Rely on God. His strength is offered to all who will but receive it.

TODAY'S THOUGHT: I would rather be Spirit-filled than calorie-filled!

Day 29

For I am in a strait betwixt two, having a desire to depart, and to be with Christ; which is far better: Nevertheless to abide in the flesh is more needful for you. PHILIPPIANS 1:23–24

Paul questioned why God had put him on earth in the first place. Being fat seemed like unnecessary torture. The diets were killers, and they didn't seem to do any good, anyway. What was the use of trying and failing over and over again? Better to never have been born.

Despair and frustration are a part of dieting. Often it seems so hopeless. Still, God has given us life as a gift. We prepare ourselves in this life for eternal life in God's presence. Now is the time we need to learn self-discipline and control. Now is the time to strive to be everything we are meant to be. Our life in the flesh is necessary, and it is up to us to make sure we take proper care of ourselves.

TODAY'S THOUGHT: I'll try my hardest to lose weight today, because I may not get another chance!

Day 30

That if thou shalt confess with thy mouth the Lord Jesus, and shalt believe in thine heart that God hath raised him from the dead, thou shalt be saved. ROMANS 10:9

Why do so many people believe that God has absolute power over life and death but doubt whether He can do anything to help them transform a small part of their own lives? Why should a few pounds of flesh be a more insurmountable obstacle than a mountain or a stone that sealed a tomb? True faith reminds us that our Lord is the Lord of the impossible. He enables us to rise above our limitations through the power of the Holy Spirit. Our God must be the Lord of the diet, too. The Lord who resurrected Jesus Christ on Easter morning will faithfully resurrect us from a tomb of obesity and flesh. Trust in God's power, for by it we are saved.

TODAY'S THOUGHT: I need Jesus to save me from me!

DAY 31

The husbandman that laboureth must be first partaker of the fruits.
2 TIMOTHY 2:6

Wendy thought she was dieting for her husband and family. She kept telling herself she was doing it for them, anyway. As the pounds melted away, however, Wendy realized something very important. No matter who she said she was doing it for, she came out the big winner. She looked better; she felt better, and she loved every minute of it. She knew she was doing something really right. She put forth a lot of sweat and tears, and she was reaping the big benefits. Not only was she dieting for her family, but she was doing it for herself, and that was a good thing. She was worth it.

TODAY'S THOUGHT: My diet is a really great decision on my part!

DAY 32

I therefore, the prisoner of the Lord, beseech you that ye walk worthy of the vocation wherewith ye are called. EPHESIANS 4:1

Rodney let himself go completely. His friends were uncomfortable when he was around. He ate constantly, and he seemed to grow larger by the day. No one knew how to talk to him about it, so they let it slide. Finally, Barb took him aside and asked him why he was destroying himself. She told him that people were losing their respect for him and couldn't understand it. In anger, Rodney told Barb it was none of her business and stormed off.

As Christians, it is other people's business when we follow paths that are not worthy of Jesus Christ. He has called us to be living examples of Himself. To be less than that is a sin. Let us try to live life in a body fit for Christ.

TODAY'S THOUGHT: Do people see Christ when they look at me?

Day 33

And whatsoever ye do, do it heartily, as to the Lord, and not unto men.
COLOSSIANS 3:23

Alice was right: Doug had been doing his diet halfway. His heart hadn't really been in it, and Alice asked him why he was even doing it at all. Now, he felt he was ready. Alice had offered the challenge, and he aimed to take her up on it. No more halfway measures: He was going to throw all his energy and commitment into losing some weight.

God wants us to mean what we say. Our yes must mean yes, and our no must mean no. Whatever we choose to do, we ought to do it fully; for God wants children with commitment and resolve, not indecision and insincerity.

TODAY'S THOUGHT: My diet is an all-or-nothing proposition!

Day 34

As the whirlwind passeth, so is the wicked no more: but the righteous is an everlasting foundation.
PROVERBS 10:25

When the group began, there were sixteen people involved. They all made a contract to lose twenty pounds by spring. When spring was less than two weeks away, the group was down to seven members. As Jean walked along the sidewalk toward the building where her group met, she noticed some small saplings bending in the stiff March breeze. Some had broken off, but a few determined little plants held on for dear life. "I'm like that," Jean thought. "Most of the others have given up, but I'm going to hang in there, no matter how stiff the challenge." Perseverance is a huge part of a successful diet. Continually ask God for commitment to your cause. He is good to give it.

TODAY'S THOUGHT: I'm determined to make it, no matter what!

Day 35

I will not leave you comfortless: I will come to you.   John 14:18

Joan was such a great friend. Almost every day she would stop by to see how things were going. Joan had been there herself. She had battled her weight for years. It was comforting to have someone around who had made it. Joan looked great. Just knowing it could be done made the whole diet easier somehow.

When we try to lose weight all by ourselves, the struggle is doubly difficult. We all need support in tough times. We can count on God's comfort when we diet. He has promised that He will never leave us comfortless. Believe in that promise. When our diets seem most futile, God will come to us.

TODAY'S THOUGHT: With the help of friends, I can lose more pounds!

Day 36

Come unto me, all ye that labour and are heavy laden, and I will give you rest.   Matthew 11:28

Sunday was "anything goes" day. Carol had decided that if she was good about sticking to her diet through the week, she would allow herself to splurge on Sunday. It made the diet so much more tolerable. Interestingly, she never really went overboard on Sunday. She ate something she really liked, but she ate a moderate amount and found herself totally satisfied.

Whenever we attempt something difficult, we need to allow ourselves a respite. It is a good thing to take a break, even from a diet. It requires self-control, but it can help us keep a healthy perspective on why we diet in the first place. Once we have rested from our fast, we can return to it renewed.

TODAY'S THOUGHT: I am tired of being heavy-ladened physically!

Day 37

Peace I leave with you, my peace I give unto you: not as the world giveth, give I unto you. Let not your heart be troubled, neither let it be afraid.   JOHN 14:27

Bill felt it was a no-win situation. If he dieted, he felt lousy because he was hungry all the time. If he broke his diet, he felt guilty. It was hard to tell which was worse, the hunger or the guilt. He wanted to trim down, but he loved to eat. He never knew that he'd suffer through so much turmoil just trying to lose weight.

Diets can really stir us up. They make us feel physically and emotionally strained. During periods of dieting, we need to find peace of mind and heart. Ask God for that peace. He promises to deliver it to those who ask Him for it. When we need it most, God gladly gives it.

TODAY'S THOUGHT: Better to have peace of mind than a piece of cake!

Day 38

For it is God which worketh in you both to will and to do of his good pleasure.   PHILIPPIANS 2:13

Stephanie got fantastic grades in algebra. All her friends were jealous of her abilities in class. Stephanie always smiled to herself. None of her friends realized that her father was a scientist who used algebra all the time. He tutored her every evening and helped her understand the problems that gave her friends such fits.

There are times when we need special help. Without it we struggle twice as hard as we really need to. God offers to help us through our diets. Allow God to work within you as you diet, and you'll be surprised how much easier it is.

TODAY'S THOUGHT: When the fat won't go away, take a moment then to pray!

Day 39

He shall feed his flock like a shepherd: he shall gather the lambs with his arm, and carry them in his bosom, and shall gently lead those that are with young.   ISAIAH 40:11

Mary blew it. She had been doing so well, then she gave in completely. In a week she gained back what had taken her a month to lose. Depressed, she called her mother for comfort. Mom was always good at that. If anyone could get her back on the right track, it was her mother. She could always trust her mother to give her sound, loving advice.

God is like that. We can trust that He will guide us along good paths. When we need someone to comfort us without condemnation, God is always there for us. He will gather us to Himself and make us ready to go on.

TODAY'S THOUGHT: I may be weak, but I'm strong enough to call on God's help!

Day 40

Though I walk in the midst of trouble, thou wilt revive me: thou shalt stretch forth thine hand against the wrath of mine enemies, and thy right hand shall save me.   PSALM 138:7

It was war! Greg looked at the bag of cookies on the table in front of him, and they almost made him cry. Why couldn't he just ignore them? It was as if they had some kind of magical spell over him. Closing his eyes didn't help. Neither did putting them in the cabinet; he still knew they were there. He was determined to resist their pull, but was he really strong enough?

When the temptations get to be too much, we need to call on the Lord. In the midst of our stiffest challenges, He will truly save us.

TODAY'S THOUGHT: I need God to save me from myself!

Day 41

For the LORD shall be thy confidence, and shall keep thy foot from being taken. PROVERBS 3:26

Norm felt drowsy, but he didn't want to stop. He only had a few miles to go to get home. Home. He began thinking about how nice it would be to get there and fall into a comfortable bed. Before he knew it, he was dropping off to sleep. He came to with a jolt as his fender scraped along the guardrail at the side of the road. Thank God for the guardrail! Without it, Norm didn't know where he'd be.

We need guardrails. They keep us from pitching off into nothingness—past the point of no return. God can be our guardrail, keeping us from indulging our appetites past reasonable limitations. Truly, He keeps us from falling.

TODAY'S THOUGHT: Food is a trap I'd rather not fall into!

Day 42

And the light shineth in darkness; and the darkness comprehended it not. JOHN 1:5

Rusty scared herself. She walked past the mirror in the dim light of dusk and thought there was a stranger in the house. How had she gotten so big? Who was she kidding? She kept telling herself that she wasn't that big, but it was so bad she didn't recognize herself in the mirror. It was like a revelation—a bright light shining through the darkness. She had to do something about her weight. Determined, she set out to lose the weight she had gained, and with God's help, she was able to do just that.

TODAY'S THOUGHT: I want to find out just how good I can look!

Day 43

When Jesus had lifted up himself, and saw none but the woman, he said unto her, Woman, where are those thine accusers? hath no man condemned thee? She said, No man, Lord. And Jesus said unto her, Neither do I condemn thee: go, and sin no more.   JOHN 8:10–11

The doctor was going to kill her. Kate had been told to lose thirty pounds over six months. For awhile she had done really well. She took off twenty in the first three months, but lately she had gained again, for a net loss of only about twelve pounds. Kate was astonished when the doctor merely encouraged her to try harder.

Christ, like the doctor, offers us no condemnation. He wants us to lose weight for our own sakes, not for His. He wants to help us, not hurt us. Take comfort in the acceptance of Jesus Christ.

TODAY'S THOUGHT: Even when I give in, I'm still a good person.

Day 44

For there is no respect of persons with God.   ROMANS 2:11

Andrea was furious. She hadn't wanted to go on the hike in the first place, and now she was falling farther and farther behind. No one would give her time to catch up. Some of them were even laughing at her. It wasn't her fault she wasn't in good physical condition. She had to carry around a lot more weight than they did. It just wasn't fair.

In this life, we don't get a lot of breaks. Just because we're overweight doesn't mean we deserve special treatment. God doesn't give preferential treatment. He wants all of His children to be the best they can possibly be. He expects us all to do our best.

TODAY'S THOUGHT: I am trying my best to please God!

Day 45

And he said to the woman, Thy faith hath saved thee; go in peace.
LUKE 7:50

God will help us as we diet, but the weight of the responsibility still lies with us. We have to really want to lose weight. God will not do it for us. Faith is the key to unlocking God's power in our lives. When we put our faith in God, He is able to lead us in new ways. He fills us with strength, courage, purpose, and the will to succeed. God has already placed those qualities in each one of us. Faith is our way of allowing God to show us how to use what we've already got. Let us remain open to God so we can succeed in losing the weight that doesn't need to be there.

TODAY'S THOUGHT: God has given me everything I need to fight fat!

Day 46

But God, who is rich in mercy, for his great love wherewith he loved us, even when we were dead in sins, hath quickened us together with Christ, (by grace ye are saved).
EPHESIANS 2:4–5

It really isn't a matter of whether God loves us more if we are thin than He does if we're fat. God loves us the same, no matter what. He loves sinners as much as He loves saints. His greatest desire, though, is for His children to be everything they can be. He wants us to desire perfection. The gluttony and selfishness that lead to obesity are not qualities of perfection. God wants us to attempt to live our lives as Jesus lived His. Let us vow to walk in a newness of life, transformed by the power of the Holy Spirit, on the road to Christlike perfection.

TODAY'S THOUGHT: God can make me better than I ever dreamed possible!

Day 47

Comfort ye, comfort ye my people, saith your God.   ISAIAH 40:1

Josh was feeling down and depressed. Nothing seemed to be working out for him. His job was a nightmare; his social life was even worse, and he was lonely. He sat alone and ate. His weight had skyrocketed. He wouldn't eat so much if he had someone to talk to. His main problem was that he just didn't have anything else to do.

Often, the most comforting thing we can hope for is someone to spend time with. Company gives us pleasure and takes our minds off eating. It is up to us to find people to spend time with when that is the only reason we sit and stuff ourselves. God sends us comfort in many ways. Seek the comfort of company.

TODAY'S THOUGHT: I'm never so tempted to cheat as when I'm alone!

Day 48

And let the peace of God rule in your hearts, to the which also ye are called in one body; and be ye thankful.   COLOSSIANS 3:15

Scott was cranky. He had been on a diet for two weeks, and it wasn't getting easier. Now his friends wanted to drag him off to some stupid prayer meeting at the church. Begrudgingly, Scott agreed to go. Before long, his mind was off of food and onto the message the pastor was delivering. Scott got caught up in praying for the needs of others, and he completely forgot about his own hunger. The time passed quickly, and Scott was surprised. His friends just smiled and told Scott that there was a lesson there for him somewhere.

When we turn our attention from ourselves to others, great things can happen.

TODAY'S THOUGHT: I want to care for others as much as I care about myself!

DAY 49

And I heard a great voice out of heaven saying, Behold, the tabernacle of God is with men, and he will dwell with them, and they shall be his people, and God himself shall be with them, and be their God.
REVELATION 21:3

Cathy decided to make a contract with God rather than a promise to herself. She vowed that she would lose weight for Him, not for any vain or selfish reason she could come up with. Somehow it was easier to do for God than it had been for herself. The pounds melted more quickly. Cathy continued her diet with regular prayer and recommitment to the promise she had made to God. Before long, Cathy had lost all the weight she set out to lose.

Our promises to God are very important. Often we can do for Him what we fail to do for ourselves. God has promised to help us whenever we need Him. He will help us lose weight.

TODAY'S THOUGHT: My diet is more than a wish; it is a promise to God.

DAY 50

Wherefore comfort yourselves together, and edify one another, even as also ye do.
1 THESSALONIANS 5:11

Joining the group was the best move she ever made. Fay had struggled alone through a dozen diets with no real success. Then she saw the notice on the church bulletin board about the group that dieted and exercised together. She was a little hesitant at first, but finally she decided to give it a try. What a difference it made! Dieting with a group was much better than dieting alone. Fay felt that God had really led her to this group. She gained so much strength from her new friends, and she was amazed at how much she was able to help others.

TODAY'S THOUGHT: A diet for two is easier to do!

DAY 51

Behold, he that keepeth Israel shall neither slumber nor sleep. The LORD is thy keeper: the LORD is thy shade upon thy right hand.

PSALM 121:4–5

The Hebrew people had great confidence in God. They believed His promises to them, and they lived their lives accordingly. No matter how difficult their situation got, the children of Israel held onto their faith. Through that faith, they were able to do amazing things.

The God of Abraham and Isaac is also the God of Jesus Christ. If we will put our faith in Him, He will enable us to do amazing things. He will allow us to lose the weight we need to lose, and He will comfort us when our diets get particularly tough. Trust in the Lord. He is watching over you.

TODAY'S THOUGHT: I'd better watch what I eat as closely as God watches me!

DAY 52

Are not two sparrows sold for a farthing? and one of them shall not fall on the ground without your Father. Fear ye not therefore, ye are of more value than many sparrows. MATTHEW 10:29, 31

Jeff was suspicious. He couldn't figure out why his friends were trying to be so helpful with his diet. What could they possibly get out of it? Whenever he was with them, they avoided talking about food, and they ate salads and cottage cheese instead of normal food. They wouldn't even have dessert. It made Jeff feel a little awkward and guilty. He couldn't believe his friends would go to so much trouble to help him out.

Some people wonder whether or not God really cares about their diet problems. The fact is, He cares about everything that is important to us. Take comfort in the fact that God cares deeply, and He will do everything He can to help you.

TODAY'S THOUGHT: God thinks I'm great, with or without weight!

DAY 53

For God sent not his Son into the world to condemn the world; but that the world through him might be saved.　　　JOHN 3:17

Guilt. Every time Liz slipped, she felt guilty. Her husband gave her such disapproving looks. She wanted to stick to her diet, but it was hard. Then, when people made her feel guilty, she got depressed, which only made her want to eat more. The more she ate, the guiltier she felt; the guiltier she felt, the more she ate. It was a vicious cycle. She wished people would be more understanding. She honestly believed that would make all the difference.

　We don't need pressure put on us by those who condemn us for not being perfect. That's why God is the perfect diet mate. He supports without condemning, and He loves us even when we fail.

TODAY'S THOUGHT: I can do wonderful things with God's support!

DAY 54

And Jesus answered and said unto her, Martha, Martha, thou art careful and troubled about many things: But one thing is needful: and Mary hath chosen that good part, which shall not be taken away from her.　　　LUKE 10:41–42

Angie brought home a new diet book each week. She had a closet full of exercisers guaranteed to take off pounds and inches. She had a cabinet full of pills, powders, and liquids bearing promises of miraculous weight loss. Cindy just shook her head. Why go to all the trouble? Losing weight wasn't going to come from anywhere except from inside the person who wanted to lose it. Desire was the main ingredient. It was too easy to get caught up in fads and fancy claims. A quiet determination to lose weight was what was really important. Angie lost a few pounds, while Cindy lost many.

TODAY'S THOUGHT: It's hard to lose weight when you have a fat head!

DAY 55

If a man therefore purge himself from these, he shall be a vessel unto honour, sanctified, and meet for the master's use, and prepared unto every good work.   2 TIMOTHY 2:21

Gary couldn't believe what he was hearing. He hadn't been selected for the mission because he was just a few pounds overweight. Harrison was trimmer, but that didn't mean he was any better as a pilot. How could they turn him down because of a few pounds?

Often being fit is determined by how trim and slim we are. It may not be fair, but it shows the value that is put on keeping in shape. God wants us to be in shape so we can enjoy this life we have been given to the fullest. He intends that we should always be ready to experience all that life has to offer. We can only do that when we take proper care of ourselves.

TODAY'S THOUGHT: I am making myself fit for life!

DAY 56

But after that the kindness and love of God our Saviour toward man appeared, not by works of righteousness which we have done, but according to his mercy he saved us, by the washing of regeneration, and renewing of the Holy Ghost.   TITUS 3:4–5

It was a miraculous metamorphosis. Darleen had lost one hundred pounds. Though everyone had encouraged her as much as possible, no one had really believed she could do it. The proof was before their eyes—Darleen looked great. Someone asked her how she had done it, and she told them that a crisis in her life had made her realize she didn't just need to lose weight, she needed to be saved from her own body. She fell in her kitchen and had not been able to get up again. Through her pain and frustration, she believed she was being taught a valuable lesson. She thanked God that He had gotten through to her before it was too late.

TODAY'S THOUGHT: Save me from being a prisoner to obesity!

Day 57

Who shall separate us from the love of Christ? shall tribulation, or distress, or persecution, or famine, or nakedness, or peril, or sword? Nay, in all these things we are more than conquerors through him that loved us.   ROMANS 8:35, 37

Christ makes us conquerors. He offers us unimaginable power through the Holy Spirit. Nothing can separate us from that love and power. That power enabled Jesus Christ to conquer death. It allowed the apostle Paul to conquer his afflictions. It allowed Peter to overcome his doubts and fears. If the Holy Spirit could do that for those great men, then why shouldn't we be able to believe that the Spirit will help us lose weight? Indeed, we can even conquer obesity through the divine power of God. Nothing can stop us from achieving our goal, because the power of God is with us.

TODAY'S THOUGHT: I will burn up calories in the fire of the Holy Spirit!

Day 58

For we have great joy and consolation in thy love, because the bowels of the saints are refreshed by thee, brother.   PHILEMON 7

Phil had a lousy self-image. He felt unwanted and unloved. He looked at himself in the mirror and saw an enormous slob. No one could love that. Dieting didn't even make sense. It was useless. Nothing would ever change.

Poor Phil honestly believed he was unloved. He had no reason to change, because he saw no hope for his future. How sad that Phil didn't know the love of God. We can proceed with our diets knowing that we are loved and that we are lovable. Just knowing that makes it all worthwhile. We draw strength from the comfort that comes from being loved. That strength ensures that we can lose the weight we want to lose.

TODAY'S THOUGHT: Special people can do anything they set their minds to, and I am a special person!

DAY 59

Judge not, and ye shall not be judged: condemn not, and ye shall not be condemned: forgive, and ye shall be forgiven. LUKE 6:37

Kelly was unbearable. She had lost thirty pounds with relative ease, so she ridiculed anyone who couldn't do it as easily as she had. Kelly wasn't being fair. Every person is different. It didn't mean that others weren't as committed or as dedicated as Kelly had been. It was frustrating to try so hard and then have Kelly make fun of you for it. Why couldn't she have a little compassion? After all, she had been obese once!

After losing weight, we should be more compassionate than anyone else. It is important to remember how hard losing weight really is. We have a wonderful opportunity to help others when we keep in mind what we've come through.

TODAY'S THOUGHT: I hope I can lose my weight without losing my sensitivity toward others!

DAY 60

And the Lord shall deliver me from every evil work, and will preserve me unto his heavenly kingdom: to whom be glory for ever and ever. Amen. 2 TIMOTHY 4:18

Wes looked at the sign on the refrigerator door: God is watching! What a thought! Everything he did was under God's watchful eye. A slight groan escaped his lips as he thought of the times he'd cheated through the week. He hoped it was worth it. Actually, Wes kind of liked the sign. It made him think, and once he got to thinking, his diet wasn't so bad. God had helped him avoid a lot of unnecessary snacks. There were worse things to have happen to you than to have God watching every move you made. Wes felt pretty confident. With God's help, he was really going to make it through this thing!

TODAY'S THOUGHT: God's steering me clear of the fat traps!

Day 61

For he is our peace, who hath made both one, and hath broken down the middle wall of partition between us; having abolished in his flesh the enmity, even the law of commandments contained in ordinances; for to make in himself of twain one new man, so making peace.

EPHESIANS 2:14–15

As wrong as it was, Rachel had to admit that being thin helped her fit in. She really wasn't a different person now that she was thin, but people surely treated her that way. It was unbelievable that people were so biased against those who were fat. Rachel sighed a prayer of thankfulness to God that He had helped her lose weight. It had been hard being on the outside. Nobody likes being ostracized. She also prayed that God might make people see how unfair it is to judge others based on their appearances. If God could help Rachel lose weight, perhaps He could change the bigotry of some concerning obesity.

TODAY'S THOUGHT: Fat or skinny, I'm the same person inside!

Day 62

And ye shall be my people, and I will be your God.

JEREMIAH 30:22

The covenant that God made was quite simple: He would be God to a group of people who would accept Him and honor Him. God's promises are always simple and straightforward. There are never strings attached. God will do everything He can to help us deal with this life. He wants to see His children happy and fulfilled. That is why He will help us when we need His comforting strength. Alone, we just don't have what it takes to make it. With God, however, there is no force on earth great enough to keep us from our goal. Remember God, and truly He will remember you in time of need.

TODAY'S THOUGHT: My willpower comes from the strongest power source around!

DAY 63

That he would grant you, according to the riches of his glory, to be strengthened with might by his Spirit in the inner man.

EPHESIANS 3:16

Herm couldn't figure out why he wasn't losing weight. He knew he wasn't eating as much as he had before he retired. When he was on the road, he ate like a horse. Now that he was home all the time, he ate a lot less. Something definitely wasn't right.

Losing weight requires much more than just changing our eating habits. We need to change our whole outlook on things. Sometimes we need to cut back on food while increasing the amount of exercise we get. Other times we need to give up certain foods altogether. We need to evaluate deep inside how we live our lives and make adjustments necessary to succeed in losing weight.

TODAY'S THOUGHT: Dieting doesn't happen on its own. It takes a conscious effort!

DAY 64

Now our Lord Jesus Christ himself, and God, even our Father, which hath loved us, and hath given us everlasting consolation and good hope through grace, comfort your hearts, and stablish you in every good word and work.

2 THESSALONIANS 2:16–17

Another diet. Carla had tried so many, and she had never come close to succeeding. She wasn't even sure why she was trying again. She knew it would be good for her to lose weight, but she felt beaten before she even began. What would make this time any different than the rest?

What makes one attempt different than others is this: confidence. We really have to believe that we can do it. It should help us immensely to know that God believes in us. He knows us better than we know ourselves, and He has equipped us with everything we need to succeed. All we have to do is learn to believe.

TODAY'S THOUGHT: What I lack in confidence, I make up for with faith!

DAY 65

Now the Lord of peace himself give you peace always by all means.
The Lord be with you all. 2 THESSALONIANS 3:16

Ted felt the material rip the moment he bent over. Funny, that never happened a few years ago. Either his clothes were all shrinking or he was filling out a bit. There was just one thing to do about it: He was going to have to lose a few pounds. He'd done it before; he could do it again. A little willpower, a little patience, and a few prayers for strength. Ted was a man who knew his God and believed He would help out. He had never doubted Him, and God had never let him down. It was nice to feel so confident about something. Dieting was easy when you were positive that God would help you work things out.

TODAY'S THOUGHT: I'm going to wear clothes I haven't fit into in years!

DAY 66

Not that we are sufficient of ourselves to think any thing as of ourselves; but our sufficiency is of God. 2 CORINTHIANS 3:5

Muriel knew she couldn't do it alone. She wasn't strong enough. Her friend Ann told her that one of her strengths was realizing she was weak. Too many of her friends tackled diets on their own and failed miserably. Well, Muriel wasn't going to make the same mistake. She wanted help from the outset.

If we realize our weaknesses and limitations, then we are better able to cope with them. God will help us to be honest with ourselves, so we can work to turn our weaknesses into strengths. Pray to God for that insight.

TODAY'S THOUGHT: What I want to eat and what I need to eat are two different things!

Day 67

Fear thou not; for I am with thee: be not dismayed; for I am thy God:
I will strengthen thee; yea, I will help thee; yea, I will uphold thee
with the right hand of my righteousness. ISAIAH 41:10

Ben was afraid to even try a diet. He never had much luck with things
that required a lot of willpower on his part. He caved in much too easily. If only someone else would make his decisions for him. He had
never been overweight when he lived at home and had his mother
around to tell him what to eat and what not to eat. Ben would be the
first one to admit that he had no self-control.

Unfortunately, we all have to learn to discipline ourselves. God
doesn't tell us what to do. He gives us complete freedom, but He will
help us have the strength to make right decisions if we ask Him to. In-
clude God, and He will make some wonderful things happen.

TODAY'S THOUGHT: True power is the ability to say no!

Day 68

For I am the LORD, I change not; therefore ye sons of Jacob are not
consumed. MALACHI 3:6

God was such a big help when Gwen began her diet, but He didn't
seem to care much anymore. Lately, Gwen's diet had become almost
intolerable. She began to wonder if God knew what she was going
through. She had prayed daily when she started her diet, and it had
gotten so easy that she really didn't need to pray all the time. Then, it
started getting harder. Why did God let that happen?

Poor Gwen never realized that God hadn't changed, but she had. She
had included God all the time at first, then she left Him out more and
more. God will help us just as much as we allow Him to. Often we are
our own, and God's, worst enemy when we take our lives out of God's
hands and put them into our own.

TODAY'S THOUGHT: God and I are dieting together!

Day 69

Ask, and it shall be given you; seek, and ye shall find; knock, and it shall be opened unto you: For every one that asketh receiveth; and he that seeketh findeth; and to him that knocketh it shall be opened.

MATTHEW 7:7–8

Barry never really believed that he'd lose weight. That was likely his problem. His heart was never in it. Whenever he got the least bit discouraged, he'd immediately give up. His friends tried to offer support, but Barry always came up with excuses for why he should give up his diet.

If we want to lose weight, we need to believe in ourselves. Self-doubt is a killer. If we lack faith in ourselves, then perhaps we can overcome it by the faith we have in God. God can fill us with a self-assurance that allows us to do almost anything we set our minds to. Push aside doubt. Be filled with the confidence of God.

TODAY'S THOUGHT: With God's help, I'll knock off a few pounds!

Day 70

The Lord is not slack concerning his promise, as some men count slackness; but is longsuffering to us-ward, not willing that any should perish, but that all should come to repentance.   2 PETER 3:9

Lois woke up from the strangest dream. She had died and gone to heaven, but when she got there, she couldn't get in. There was an extremely narrow hallway that each person had to pass through before he or she could enter heaven. Try as she might, Lois couldn't get through the passageway because she was so large. Before, she had doubted that she could lose weight. Now, she found a new motivation. She believed God had broken through her excuses to tell her how important it was for her to lose. Never once did she believe that God would keep her out of heaven because of her weight, but she realized that her weight already kept her from enjoying life the way God intended it to be.

TODAY'S THOUGHT: Life is great when you carry less weight!

Day 71

Thou shalt make thy prayer unto him, and he shall hear thee, and thou shalt pay thy vows.   JOB 22:27

Gary took time every morning to pray about his diet. Some days he awoke frustrated that he wasn't losing weight. Other days he awoke with cravings, afraid he wouldn't be able to withstand temptation. Still other mornings he just wanted to thank God that he'd come so far. God helped make the diet bearable. Every time Gary found himself feeling ready to give up, a quick prayer to God gave him the willpower to go on.

The power of God is a wonderful thing. We cannot comprehend how much God does for us when we call upon His name. Rest assured that God is with you in all you do. . .even in your diet.

TODAY'S THOUGHT: The more time you pray, the less you can weigh!

Day 72

The righteous cry, and the LORD heareth, and delivereth them out of all their troubles.   PSALM 34:17

Pat lay crying in bed. It was so hard. It seemed that for every three pounds she lost, she immediately gained two back. She really wanted to lose weight, but she felt so weak in the face of temptation. Wasn't there anything that could help her?

Pat fell asleep that night with a prayer on her lips. Strangely, she felt a wonderful peace the next morning. The battle was truly tough, but she was once more ready to face it. God didn't take away the struggle, but He was able to give Pat just what she needed to carry on. That is the wonder of our God.

TODAY'S THOUGHT: I'll keep fighting fat until I'm fit!

DAY 73

And seek not ye what ye shall eat, or what ye shall drink, neither be ye of doubtful mind.   LUKE 12:29

Clyde was so infuriating! Every time his wife suggested that he go on a diet, he came up with some excuse. Most of the time he just said that diets weren't healthy. He was afraid he would do more harm than good. Clyde knew it was just a dodge. He didn't want to lose weight, and he saw no reason why anyone should want to push him. That all changed when he landed in the hospital with a heart attack brought on because his body simply couldn't carry the weight Clyde contained. Clyde no longer questioned what was right. Instead of doubting the intelligence of dieting, he wondered why he had ever been so stupid as to resist it. Sometimes God needs to let us know through crisis what we will not hear normally.

TODAY'S THOUGHT: If it's a choice between dieting or dying, I think I'll diet!

DAY 74

And the peace of God, which passeth all understanding, shall keep your hearts and minds through Christ Jesus.   PHILIPPIANS 4:7

Jessica was doubtful, at first. She really didn't believe Mindy when she said the church would be a big help during her diet. Mindy had taken her to see the pastor, and they had told him that they were dieting. She felt silly at first, but the pastor asked regularly how they were doing, and Jessica liked that. It made her feel that what she was doing was important and a good thing. Other members of the church mentioned how good the dieters were looking. Before long, Jessica found that she enjoyed the dieting because she enjoyed the reactions of the church people and didn't want to let them down. Mindy was right: The church helped a lot.

TODAY'S THOUGHT: Sharing the load of dieting makes the burden lighter!

DAY 75

For God hath not given us the spirit of fear; but of power, and of love, and of a sound mind.   2 TIMOTHY 1:7

Brenda decided it was time to lose weight, and she did it. Peggy struggled a little bit more, but she lost the pounds she wanted to, also. Tracy wondered why everyone else seemed to do so well, while she did so poorly. Maybe something was wrong with her! Maybe she couldn't lose weight. The more she thought about it, the more frightened she became.

Often our minds turn out to be our worst enemies when we try to diet. We can alarm ourselves needlessly. Everyone diets differently, and everyone receives different results. There is no place for fear and doubting in dieting. What we need is perseverance and faith that God will help us.

TODAY'S THOUGHT: I have a very skinny spirit!

DAY 76

And being fully persuaded that, what he had promised, he was able also to perform.   ROMANS 4:21

Jesus Christ turned water to wine; He walked on the water and calmed the sea. He cured many diseases and cast out demons. He conquered death for His friend Lazarus and for Himself. He promises that He will be with us and that His power is ours as we try to be the people God created us to be. How, then, can we doubt that He will help us when we need to lose weight? Are not the pounds of our flesh within His scope of power? Cannot the chosen Son of God do such a small miracle in our lives as to give us the determination we need to conquer fat? This He can and will do, and much more, if we will but believe.

TODAY'S THOUGHT: "More" brought about my distress; help me, Lord, to live by "less"!

DAY 77

Set your affection on things above, not on things on the earth.
COLOSSIANS 3:2

The smells from the cafeteria were more than Blanche could take. Not that the cafeteria food was anything to write home about, but when she was on a diet, almost anything smelled good! She grabbed her jacket and headed out the door. Immediately, the fresh fall air erased the cafeteria smells. The sky was a deep blue, and the white clouds lazily drifted by. The sun was out, the birds were singing, and everything was right with the world. Blanche spent her lunch hour just strolling through God's splendor. Before she knew it, her hunger had passed, and she was ready to tackle the afternoon. The glory of God had lifted her above her earthly passions, and she was grateful.

TODAY'S THOUGHT: There's much more to life than lunch!

DAY 78

Thou wilt keep him in perfect peace, whose mind is stayed on thee: because he trusteth in thee. ISAIAH 26:3

Bud believed his doctor really did have his best interests in mind. Bud wouldn't have dieted if anyone else had told him he should, but his doctor was a little more serious. Bud kept to the diet because he felt it was the right thing to do. Trust was a big factor in making everything work.

Trust is a big factor in anything we try to do. Giants of the Christian faith were able to do such great things because they trusted that the Lord was with them. We, perhaps not giants of the faith, need to rest assured that we can trust God and that He will do everything He can to help us lose weight.

TODAY'S THOUGHT: The only thing God will let down is my weight!

Day 79

When thou liest down, thou shalt not be afraid: yea, thou shalt lie down, and thy sleep shall be sweet.   PROVERBS 3:24

Janice remembered long, sleepless nights where she tossed and turned, feeling guilty that she had cheated on her diet or merely crying because she was so enormous. Thank God those nights were long gone. Being fat was not just a physical trauma but an emotional and mental one, as well. She never realized how much her peace of mind was dependent on her waistline until she took off the excess weight. Now she had wonderful nights and wonderful days. Her life was transformed. God had been so good to her. She felt she'd been given a new life. This time she was determined to take care of it.

TODAY'S THOUGHT: Losing weight promises a new lease on life!

Day 80

The Lord knoweth how to deliver the godly out of temptations, and to reserve the unjust unto the day of judgment to be punished.
2 PETER 2:9

Woody had a weird dream. His hands and arms got so flabby that he couldn't reach out to pick anything up anymore. Before him stood a long table filled with marvelous things to eat, but he was unable to take anything. He woke up sweat soaked and shuddering. It seemed so real! He caught a glimpse of himself in the dresser mirror as he sat alone in the night. He was getting awfully plump. Maybe somebody was trying to tell him something. He was no fool. They say that God moves in mysterious ways, and maybe that was true. No reason to push the old luck. Tomorrow the diet would begin!

TODAY'S THOUGHT: I remember when my eyes could be bigger than my stomach!

DAY 81

I can do all things through Christ which strengtheneth me.

PHILIPPIANS 4:13

Jerome stepped up in front of the huge audience. Not too long ago, Jerome wouldn't have been caught dead speaking publicly. All that changed when he found he had something to talk about. Jesus Christ had changed his life, and he wanted the whole world to know. Jerome truly believed that anything was possible for him now that Jesus Christ was the center of his life.

That same confidence can be ours when we turn our lives over to Jesus. Christ transforms us and enables us to do things that we doubted were possible before. Trust the Lord to help you lose weight and watch the miracle begin.

TODAY'S THOUGHT: I become more spiritually as I become less physically!

DAY 82

And he said unto me, My grace is sufficient for thee: for my strength is made perfect in weakness. Most gladly therefore will I rather glory in my infirmities, that the power of Christ may rest upon me.

2 CORINTHIANS 12:9

There are times when the hunger pangs get to be almost unbearable. A person gets shaky; she feels weak-kneed and light-headed. It almost feels like an illness. Hunger makes us aware of how weak we really are. A person who is hungry is a person who is humble.

It is good for us to realize that we need help—that we are not always able to stand on our own two feet. In those times of weakness, we learn to rely on the true strength: the power of Jesus Christ. Christ comes to us in our moments of weakness to strengthen and support us. Praise God that He never lets us fail for very long.

TODAY'S THOUGHT: Hunger makes me weak; losing weight makes me strong!

Day 83

Let us hold fast the profession of our faith without wavering; (for he is faithful that promised).   HEBREWS 10:23

Kelly believed God would help her. At least, she wanted to believe that God would help. Sometimes she wasn't so sure. She'd begin to doubt, then fear would set in, and she'd comfort herself with a bowl of ice cream or a chocolate bar. Then she'd get mad at herself; she'd pray for help once more, and the whole cycle would start again. If only she could stay convinced that God was with her to give her strength. Kelly knew it wasn't God's fault that she kept giving in. It was her own wavering. Perhaps Kelly's prayer should have been for strength of faith, rather than strength of diet willpower.

TODAY'S THOUGHT: I don't think God will help me lose weight; I know it!

Day 84

For then shalt thou lift up thy face without spot; yea, thou shalt be stedfast, and shalt not fear.   JOB 11:15

What a marvelous feeling, being able to stand up in front of the diet group and telling them she had lost forty-four pounds! Marcie never thought she'd see the day. She remembered all the times when, with great embarrassment, she'd had to confess that she was not even close to her goal. Those days were behind her. All the doubts and guilt were over. The groups had been a great help, too, as God had been. Her faith was a large reason that she was able to stay with it as well as she did. Praise God, everything worked out. She held her head high and shared her great news with the group who had helped her so much.

TODAY'S THOUGHT: Doubting never helps get things done!

DAY 85

He that overcometh shall inherit all things; and I will be his God, and he shall be my son.   REVELATION 21:7

Chris thought he was going to die. Why did the gym teacher make the fat kids run track? It wasn't humane. His pulse was pounding so hard, he thought his eyes might pop out. The finish line looked a million miles away. It wasn't worth it. Somehow he had to lose some of his excess baggage. Nobody could go through life feeling as bad as he presently felt.

We need to overcome our weight problems. Life is not meant to be a struggle but a blessed gift from God. If we will work to be overcomers, then God will bless our efforts and carry us over the finish line.

TODAY'S THOUGHT: With each pound I drop, I move faster toward my goal!

DAY 86

Surely he shall deliver thee from the snare of the fowler, and from the noisome pestilence.   PSALM 91:3

Bert woke up in a cold sweat. He had dreamed that he was lying on a beach when suddenly the sand began to shift, and he felt himself being sucked downward. Try as he might, he couldn't twist or turn out of the trap. Every way he moved, the sand gave way. He realized that the only reason he was sinking was due to his weight. The more he fought, the deeper he sank. As the sand closed in over his head, he woke up. Quietly, he prayed that the Lord might rescue him from his prison of flesh. Immediately, he was filled with a spirit of sacrifice and commitment equal to the diet that lay before him.

TODAY'S THOUGHT: Without a doubt, I'll win this bout!

DAY 87

*Therefore I say unto you, What things soever ye desire, when ye pray,
believe that ye receive them, and ye shall have them.*

MARK 11:24

Abby knew that God hadn't lost her weight for her, but He sure helped
her be able to lose it. When she felt most like giving up, He encouraged her and gave her the will to go on. When she was most tempted
to break her diet, He reminded her of how important it was to stick
with it. When the pounds began to fall, He filled her with a deep joy
that insured she would continue. She never forgot to pray, whether it
was for help, for strength, or for thanksgiving. Abby hadn't lost the
weight all by herself. God helped more than she could ever know.

TODAY'S THOUGHT: I'm glad that I'm a loser. . .of weight!

DAY 88

God is our refuge and strength, a very present help in trouble.

PSALM 46:1

Barb hated it when her husband went away on business trips. He was
her conscience when it came to watching what she ate. Besides, when
she was lonely she had the tendency to eat to compensate. It was so
much harder to diet when he went away.

It is good to know that we have a refuge and strength that never
goes on vacation. God is ever with us, and He will help us whenever
we need Him. When the temptations are the greatest, then we can be
confident that God will be the strongest.

TODAY'S THOUGHT: I will turn to God when my diet gets too tough!

DAY 89

But let him ask in faith, nothing wavering. For he that wavereth is like a wave of the sea driven with the wind and tossed.　　　JAMES 1:6

Sybil couldn't understand why Bev kept praying about her diet. It seemed so silly. Sybil was a good Christian, but she didn't bother talking about such trivial things with God. God had much better things to do than watch people lose weight, didn't He? Still, Bev seemed to be doing much better on her diet than Sybil was. Bev didn't struggle with temptation as much, and she was much better at saying no when she was offered rich, fattening foods. Maybe Bev had something. Her prayers were obviously a help to her, and Sybil had nothing to lose but her weight. Sybil decided to ask Bev for some guidance.

TODAY'S THOUGHT: Too much doubt rules weight loss out!

DAY 90

The name of the LORD is a strong tower: the righteous runneth into it, and is safe.　　　PROVERBS 18:10

Every few weeks or so, Ellen would go off by herself to her grandmother's farm for a day alone. She would fast for the entire day, and each time hunger would overtake her, she would pause to pray to God. She thanked Him for providing her with food and sustenance through the week. She thanked Him for her life in a country where she was free to do what she wanted to do. She thanked Him that she didn't have to struggle day to day for survival. The times on the farm meant so much to her. Ellen found great strength in those times when hunger made her feel so weak. It was good to take time to be thankful.

TODAY'S THOUGHT: I'll try not to think of what I don't have but what I do have!

Day 91

Fear not: for I am with thee: I will bring thy seed from the east, and
gather thee from the west. ISAIAH 43:5

It didn't look like it was going to work out. Becky wanted to lose a few
pounds before the dance. It wasn't any big deal, but that made it worse.
She'd had almost six weeks, and in that time she hadn't lost any
weight at all. She kept telling herself she had plenty of time, but time
had slipped away. Now it was too late, and she felt terrible. Why had
she been so stupid? Why hadn't she taken it more seriously? Not only
did she feel bad because she was overweight, but she also felt guilty
and hopeless. Somehow she had to learn to knuckle down and stick to
what she needed to do. With God's help, maybe she could.

TODAY'S THOUGHT: Today I lose weight; tomorrow's too late!

Day 92

And they that know thy name will put their trust in thee: for thou, LORD,
hast not forsaken them that seek thee. PSALM 9:10

It was nice to see that the church cared so much about the ladies' group
who dieted together. At the annual church planning board dinner, it was
suggested that a low-calorie menu be offered. Dieting was so much
easier when other people understood and cooperated with you. It was
gratifying to be supported by the church as if by one's own family.
God had been good to the ladies of the church.

God's love should be apparent in our churches. The church should
be a place where we know we will be affirmed and supported. God
never forsakes His children, and His children should be careful not to
forsake each other.

TODAY'S THOUGHT: No matter what, I'm not on this diet alone!

Day 93

For I the LORD thy God will hold thy right hand, saying unto thee,
Fear not; I will help thee. ISAIAH 41:13

When Jenny was young, her mother used to hold her hand whenever
Jenny was afraid or worried. Just the feel of her mother's hand in hers
gave her strength and courage. There were days when Jenny wished her
mom were close enough to hold her hand again, but she lived hundreds
of miles away. She especially wanted her mother's support now that she
was dieting. Whenever things got particularly tough, she would close
her eyes to say a short prayer. As she prayed, she imagined her hand in
Jesus' hand, and she felt a wonderful peace and comfort. That image
gave Jenny all the strength she needed.

TODAY'S THOUGHT: I'm never too heavy for God to pick up!

Day 94

These things I have spoken unto you, that in me ye might have peace.
In the world ye shall have tribulation: but be of good cheer; I have
overcome the world. JOHN 16:33

Leo wanted to remember how tough it was. He'd lost the weight, but
he never wanted to get back into the poor shape he'd recently been in.
It would be way too easy to fall back into bad habits, thinking that the
battle was won once for all time. It was nice to have succeeded. But
Leo planned to make sure his success lasted a good, long time.

It is nice to overcome obesity, but it is an ongoing battle. We should
ally ourselves with the one true conqueror: Jesus Christ. With Christ's
help, we can continue to triumph over our weight problems. He grants
not only peace, but power to overcome any obstacle.

TODAY'S THOUGHT: If we empty our plate, we won't lose our weight!

Day 95

Wait on the LORD: be of good courage, and he shall strengthen thine heart: wait, I say, on the LORD.   PSALM 27:14

Kerri wished she could lose weight just a little bit faster. She really didn't have anything to complain about. Since she started her diet, she had consistently lost. There were days, though, when she simply got tired of dieting. She doubted whether she was ever going to lose the weight she wanted to lose. At those times, she turned to God for encouragement. Talking to the Lord always made Kerri feel better. She really believed that He knew what she was going through. If God could be patient with her when she complained about her diet, she figured she could be more patient as she attempted to lose weight.

TODAY'S THOUGHT: Without patience, I'll never lose weight!

Day 96

Therefore I take pleasure in infirmities, in reproaches, in necessities, in persecutions, in distresses for Christ's sake: for when I am weak, then am I strong.   2 CORINTHIANS 12:10

Having to diet was like having a bad rash. It was almost impossible to ignore, and it never went away. It was a real test of will not to give in when the stomach started growling. More than anything, he ate regularly, just not as much as he was used to. He always prided himself on being a strong person. His diet was proving otherwise. He was short-tempered and cranky. As hard as it was, he had to admit he needed help. He prayed for God to strengthen him through his diet. With God's help, he felt he might just make it.

TODAY'S THOUGHT: I'm stronger than my stomach gives me credit for being!

Day 97

Wherefore take unto you the whole armour of God, that ye may be able to withstand in the evil day, and having done all, to stand.

EPHESIANS 6:13

Even the mightiest warrior of old was not foolish enough to enter battle without protection. Strength must be tempered with common sense. When we wage war on fat, we need to be well equipped for the fray. If we give something up, we need to have something to replace it with. Jesus proposed that we should not live by bread only but upon the Word of God. We can protect ourselves from temptation by faith. God will fight our battle alongside us. With Christ, we become an invincible army. We can carry on in the strength of the Spirit, which will allow us to conquer our weight and fears. With Christ comes true power.

TODAY'S THOUGHT: With Jesus' might, my fat I'll fight!

Day 98

The righteous also shall hold on his way, and he that hath clean hands shall be stronger and stronger.

JOB 17:9

Mort juggled his folder of papers, his coffee, and his sweet roll. It seemed as though Mort couldn't go anywhere without his hands full of food. Even now, as he rushed toward an important meeting, he fed his face. As he rounded the corner, a great gust of wind took him by surprise, ripping the folder from his hands. The sheets of his report flew off in many directions as he watched helplessly, sweet roll in hand. Looking at the messy roll clutched in his fingers, he silently swore to cut out all the snacks. Not only were they ruining his body, but now they jeopardized his job. It just wasn't worth it.

TODAY'S THOUGHT: I don't want my greatest skill to be my ability to eat!

Day 99

Not that I speak in respect of want: for I have learned, in whatsoever state I am, therewith to be content.   PHILIPPIANS 4:11

Sam remembered the POW camp he had spent six years in. Whenever he began to feel sorry for himself as he dieted, he remembered the time in his life when he really had something to be upset about. Dieting was nothing compared to what he had suffered. It humbled him a little. He gained great strength from the memory. God had gotten him through the war, so he knew God could get him through the diet. As long as he had the memory of all he had come through before, he knew he could make it through anything else that came his way.

TODAY'S THOUGHT: God brings me through every situation, whether large or small.

Day 100

I will lift up mine eyes unto the hills, from whence cometh my help. My help cometh from the LORD, which made heaven and earth.   PSALM 121:1–2

Sonya was just about to dip into the ice cream when her doorbell rang. Guiltily, she threw the container into the freezer and slammed the door. Rushing to the hallway, she opened the door and found her sister standing there. Time after time, her sister showed up when she was most needed. Sonya couldn't believe the number of times her sister had been there to help her resist temptation. Sonya felt God was really watching out for her. Whenever her own strength gave out, God sent someone along who could strengthen her. Relieved, she let her sister in and told her the service she had just performed.

TODAY'S THOUGHT: Strength comes from unexpected places when our own strength gives out!

Day 101

But they that wait upon the LORD shall renew their strength; they shall mount up with wings as eagles; they shall run, and not be weary; and they shall walk, and not faint. ISAIAH 40:31

Kip was amazed at how easily he took the stairs. When his kids had begged him to climb to the top of the Statue of Liberty with them, he had squirmed. He remembered what a labor it had been when he was fat. He knew that he never would have made it before. Instead of a painful trauma, he found the climb a relative breeze. Thank God he had been able to lose the weight. It was the best move he ever made. It had been tough, but Kip had relied heavily on God to help him out. While he had been dieting, he had needed God's strength. Now that he was thin, God let him use his own strength once again.

TODAY'S THOUGHT: Food gives us temporary strength. God gives us strength forever!

Day 102

But we are not of them who draw back unto perdition; but of them that believe to the saving of the soul. HEBREWS 10:39

Darren felt bad withdrawing from the group, but he had to. The other three men kept cheating on their diets, and that was no help at all. Each time they gave in to temptation, Darren asked himself why he tried so hard when everyone else quit. Darren needed strength and support, not more temptation. At least on his own he stood a fighting chance. Darren prayed for guidance. Dieting was hard enough without other people making it harder.

We need to attach ourselves to those who are serious and committed to losing weight. God will help us have all the strength we need to stay on our diets.

TODAY'S THOUGHT: The weight that I've lost was of minimal cost!

Day 103

Behold also the ships, which though they be so great, and are driven of fierce winds, yet are they turned about with a very small helm, whithersoever the governor listeth.   JAMES 3:4

David Gregory spoke to groups all over the country. He believed that faith could help people achieve all their goals. He spoke to grossly overweight people, and it had been his faith that had brought him through. Often people would skeptically confront him as to how he really lost all his weight. His answer never varied. When asked, he would produce a tiny pewter cross from his pocket. All his success, all his power, all his wealth were nothing compared to the strength of that small symbol. The power of the cross of Christ is unequalled.

TODAY'S THOUGHT: With each little loss of weight, I make a greater gain!

Day 104

Trust ye in the LORD for ever: for in the LORD JEHOVAH is everlasting strength.   ISAIAH 26:4

Lettuce! Celery! Low-fat cottage cheese! Ugh! It never got any more interesting. The same old bland foods got tiresome after awhile. Debbie thought she would go crazy before long. She knew what she was doing was a good thing. She really wanted to lose weight. She wanted to look and feel great. Sometimes she didn't know whether it was going to pay off. She believed that God was happy with her desire to lose weight. She trusted that He would help her. Often it was only the strength she received from trying to please God that kept her going. She was thankful that God gave her that kind of strength.

TODAY'S THOUGHT: The only thing I'll give up is being fat!

Day 105

Is any among you afflicted? let him pray. Is any merry? let him sing psalms.   JAMES 5:13

Bill kept telling June to ask God for help. June couldn't quite bring herself to do it. Prayer was for weaklings. Only people who couldn't handle life prayed. June would rather struggle by on her own than rely on a crutch. False pride is a sad affliction. People who feel that they are strong enough to handle every situation of life only fool themselves. Everyone is weak at some point in her life. The truly strong person is the one who acknowledges her weakness and has the wisdom to turn to God for help.

TODAY'S THOUGHT: More time in prayer means less time to eat!

Day 106

And who is he that will harm you, if ye be followers of that which is good?   1 PETER 3:13

Kim's mother felt so sorry for her. She remembered what it was like to be overweight. All the other children were so cruel. She could still feel the sting of all the nicknames people had put on her. Now Kim was suffering the same indignities. Her mother hoped she could get Kim on a diet, if for no other reason than to keep Kim's classmates from taunting her so mercilessly. Just taking steps to correct the problem made it easier to take. The insults didn't hurt so much after the problem was taken care of. Together they would lose the weight. With God's help, time would heal the wounds of unkind words.

TODAY'S THOUGHT: I will put all my excess weight behind me!

Day 107

But as many as received him, to them gave he power to become the sons of God, even to them that believe on his name.   JOHN 1:12

Corey had to admit that his friends were making better progress than he was. He just wasn't disciplined enough. His friends didn't seem to have nearly as much trouble with discipline. When he asked them why, they all just grinned and told him to pray about it. Finally, it dawned on him what they were talking about. Corey wasn't much of a Christian, but he wasn't stupid, either. His friends obviously had something he needed and wanted. If God could do so much to help them, then Corey believed He would do it for him, also. By receiving the truth of Christ, Corey was given all the strength needed to succeed in his diet.

TODAY'S THOUGHT: God is ready to help me lose weight!

Day 108

Submit yourselves therefore to God. Resist the devil, and he will flee from you.   JAMES 4:7

Grace was surprised. The hostess had offered her dessert, and she had declined without even the slightest pang of remorse. Dessert had always been Grace's favorite type of food. Giving up dessert had been the worst part of her diet. Now, though, she found that she had declined without really caring. What a breakthrough! She felt she had a fighting chance. She had resisted temptation so long that it wasn't tempting any longer. Grace felt stronger than at any other point in her diet. Thank God, she was going to make it, after all!

TODAY'S THOUGHT: The more I turn down, the more my weight goes down!

Day 109

Wherefore let him that thinketh he standeth take heed lest he fall.
1 CORINTHIANS 10:12

Peter dressed for the dinner. His friends tried to tell him he shouldn't go, but he ignored them. He'd been doing great on his diet. He was in total control. He knew there would be wonderful and exotic food where he was going, but he could handle it. Too bad he forgot that when he got there. The temptation was too great for him. Before he realized what was happening, he was stuffed. In one day, he blew a couple of weeks of hard work.

We can't afford to get cocky when we diet. Each day is a new struggle all its own. Ask God for daily help. Avoid situations where temptation prevails. The Lord will be sure to help you whenever you let Him.

TODAY'S THOUGHT: I will steer clear of calorie traps!

Day 110

Then he answered and spake unto me, saying, This is the word of the LORD unto Zerubbabel, saying, Not by might, nor by power, but by my spirit, saith the LORD of hosts.
ZECHARIAH 4:6

Curtis liked to think he could do everything on his own. He often told friends that he didn't need anybody else; he was fine all by himself. On those rare occasions when Curt was feeling down and in need of a friend's support, he usually found himself alone. Everyone figured he really didn't need anyone else, and so he was lonely.

No matter how strong or powerful or talented we might be, we all need the support of friends. Our greatest friend is, of course, Jesus Christ. We need never feel alone when we have the Spirit of the Lord with us. Accept the helping hand of the Lord, and find out what real strength is all about.

TODAY'S THOUGHT: Let me lose not only weight, but also false pride!

Day 111

Jesus answered, Thou couldest have no power at all against me, except it were given thee from above: therefore he that delivered me unto thee hath the greater sin.　　　　　JOHN 19:11

How much easier our lives would be if we could quit fighting the fact that all power comes from God. We want control of our own lives, and we like to think we can stand on our own two feet. The reality of the matter is that we have received everything we have from the Lord. He has given us our abilities and talents; He has given us our resources, and He gives us our opportunities. The truly strong person is she who understands that God is the source of all power. If we want the power to diet, it can come to us only through the Lord God Almighty, who loves His children and offers them everything they need.

TODAY'S THOUGHT: God is greater than my desire to eat!

Day 112

But speaking the truth in love, may grow up into him in all things, which is the head, even Christ: From whom the whole body fitly joined together and compacted by that which every joint supplieth, according to the effectual working in the measure of every part, maketh increase of the body unto the edifying of itself in love.　　　EPHESIANS 4:15–16

Peak efficiency: That is what God intended for the human body. The human body is an intricate, delicate, but powerful machine finely crafted and capable of amazing feats. The only way the body can work properly the way God intended is if we take good care of it. It should not be burdened with excessive weight, nor should it be abused by improper diet. If we will endeavor to take good care of our bodies, we will experience the joy of living the way God intended for us all.

TODAY'S THOUGHT: I am a marvelous creation of God worth taking care of!

DAY 113

*O God, thou art terrible out of thy holy places: the God of Israel is he
that giveth strength and power unto his people. Blessed be God.*

PSALM 68:35

Theo knew the power of God. He had seen it in the birth of his daughter. He had felt it when his father had died. He had witnessed it many times in the glorious creation of nature. Theo had no doubt about the power of God. He had worked in forestry for his entire life. He had flown through thunderstorms where lightning splintered huge trees and set forests blazing. The power of God was both a wonderful and a terrifying thing. Theo had no doubt that there was nothing beyond the power of God. The God of all creation could handle his diet. He had no question in his mind. Strength such as God's was a good thing to have on his side!

TODAY'S THOUGHT: With God on my side, my fat doesn't stand a chance!

DAY 114

*Moreover when ye fast, be not, as the hypocrites, of a sad countenance:
for they disfigure their faces, that they may appear unto men to fast.
Verily I say unto you, They have their reward.*   MATTHEW 6:16

Everyone knew enough to stay out of Kevin's way when he was on a diet. The man became a raving lunatic. He couldn't get along with anybody. Connie felt he acted that way just to let everyone know he was on a diet. Then, when he gave up on it, nobody had the nerve to suggest he give it another try. It was his way of justifying not having to diet. Connie just wished he'd quit putting on such performances; it made everyone else miserable.

Our diets need to be our business unless we turn to others for help. We diet for the wrong reasons if all we want is sympathy or attention. God will give strength to those who are sincere, but He is unable to help those who really don't want help.

TODAY'S THOUGHT: My diet will not become a burden to anyone else!

DAY 115

But the God of all grace, who hath called us unto his eternal glory by Christ Jesus, after that ye have suffered a while, make you perfect, stablish, strengthen, settle you.   1 PETER 5:10

Cliff felt content. He felt good about the diet. He knew it was time to do something, so it didn't feel like such a great struggle. He prayed for God's help, and he felt God's presence with him. Sure, there would be unpleasantness, as there was whenever a sacrifice was involved, but it would all be well worth it. The prospect of being healthy and trim was very appealing to him. Cliff had confidence that God would bless him with strength, courage, and peace. With that kind of assurance, how could he go wrong?

TODAY'S THOUGHT: If God will give me everything I really need, how can I help but lose weight?

DAY 116

Another parable put he forth unto them, saying, The kingdom of heaven is like to a grain of mustard seed, which a man took, and sowed in his field: Which indeed is the least of all seeds: but when it is grown, it is the greatest among herbs, and becometh a tree, so that the birds of the air come and lodge in the branches thereof.   MATTHEW 13:31–32

All too often, people tackle diets that are too big for them. They try to give up everything at once, hoping to lose a huge amount of weight in a short period of time. Usually, that won't work. We should learn that the greatest successes come in small steps. We need to set modest goals that we can handle, so we don't get discouraged. God blesses our small efforts, for they are usually the most sincere and realistic. Ask God's guidance, and He will grant you exactly the right amount of strength you need to triumph.

TODAY'S THOUGHT: Giving up a little at a time will keep me from giving up altogether!

Day 117

*Who is weak, and I am not weak? who is offended, and I burn not?
If I must needs glory, I will glory of the things which concern mine
infirmities.*   2 Corinthians 11:29–30

If there was one thing to respect Cynthia for, it was her humility. She
was very talented, but she knew well what she could do and what she
couldn't. She was never shy about asking for help when she needed it,
and she never tried to make people think she could do things she could
not. It was nice to see someone who could admit her weaknesses without being defensive or insecure. When Cynthia had dieted, she openly
admitted that she relied heavily on God for strength and encouragement. It was a real inspiration to others to find someone who gained
strength from being honest about weakness.

TODAY'S THOUGHT: It is more important to be strong of heart than
strong of body!

Day 118

*Thou hast thrust sore at me that I might fall: but the LORD helped me.
The LORD is my strength and song, and is become my salvation.*
                                               Psalm 118:13–14

Going home to Mother's was murder on the diet. Stacy dreaded it. She
knew the minute she walked in, her mother would ask her why she
wasn't eating right, and then, for the next week, her mother would
shove fattening, although delicious, dishes in front of her face. Going
home required a double measure of strength. At those times, Stacy had
to pray doubly hard. Sometimes it worked, sometimes she gave in. In
the end, though, Stacy was glad to have God to turn to. Once back in
her own apartment, He gave her all the resolve she needed to get right
back on her diet. Truly, the Lord was her strength and her salvation.

TODAY'S THOUGHT: I need saving from that which I would devour!

Day 119

Fear thou not; for I am with thee: be not dismayed; for I am thy God: I will strengthen thee; yea, I will help thee; yea, I will uphold thee with the right hand of my righteousness. ISAIAH 41:10

The evening was the worst. About an hour before bedtime, Eleanor would begin to get cravings. The worst possible thing to do would be to eat right before bed. Sometimes her stomach would growl so much that she thought she would wake up the neighborhood. On those occasions, Eleanor asked God for a little quick relief and went straight to bed. Better that than to pig out and feel lousy the rest of the night and guilty all the following day!

God can grant us blessed relief from the whinings of the stomach. He can take our mind off our stomachs and give us the strength to say no!

TODAY'S THOUGHT: The waistline won't grow if I learn to say no!

Day 120

Take my yoke upon you, and learn of me; for I am meek and lowly in heart: and ye shall find rest unto your souls. For my yoke is easy, and my burden is light. MATTHEW 11:29–30

The most impressive thing about Laura was that no one realized she was on her diet. She never complained. She never made a big deal about what she could and couldn't eat. She never whined around or moped, hoping someone would ask her what was the matter. She just quietly, patiently lost weight. The rest of the women in the office were astonished. Laura made it seem so easy. Laura just smiled at all their comments, content to know that God had rallied her spirits and helped her get by.

TODAY'S THOUGHT: During my diet, I'll smile even when I feel like crying!

DAY 121

*Forasmuch then as Christ hath suffered for us in the flesh, arm your-
selves likewise with the same mind: for he that hath suffered in the
flesh hath ceased from sin; that he no longer should live the rest of his
time in the flesh to the lusts of men, but to the will of God.*

1 PETER 4:1–2

Barney knew he could lose weight. He'd given up cigarettes, and that
was the hardest thing he'd ever had to do. If he could do away with cigarettes, he was positive he could lose weight. A friend had once told him
that if he was suffering, he knew he was on the right track. Nothing
worth doing came easy. Barney asked God for strength as he set about
losing weight. When he felt he was suffering the most, that's when he
relied most heavily on God. A little suffering never hurt anyone, especially when it was done in order to attain good health.

TODAY'S THOUGHT: I suffer now so that I can enjoy the rest of my life!

DAY 122

Wherefore lift up the hands which hang down, and the feeble knees.
HEBREWS 12:12

Monica hated evenings that she had to spend alone. When she was
with friends, she felt so much stronger. She put forth all her energy to
have a good time when she went out. On the nights she stayed home,
however, she just didn't have the strength to put on a happy front.
Dieting was so much more difficult without help from friends.

It is good to know that God is ever with us. On those occasions
when there is no one around to help us, we can turn to God for
strength and endurance. He helps us pick ourselves up and continue
on our way. He strengthens feeble knees and lifts hands that hang
down.

TODAY'S THOUGHT: My energy comes from a source other than food!

DAY 123

Confess your faults one to another, and pray one for another, that ye may be healed. The effectual fervent prayer of a righteous man availeth much.   JAMES 5:16

The best idea the group ever had was to pray for one another. Every Monday morning, they got together for exercise and a Bible study. They talked about their diets and how things were going, and they had to announce publicly what their weight was and how much they had lost or gained. Then, they promised to pray for one another, and they swapped telephone numbers so they could give a call of encouragement through the week. It was a wonderful system, and it helped so much to know you weren't dieting alone. The power of a well-meant prayer was amazing. It made dieting much easier.

TODAY'S THOUGHT: A prayer a day keeps the flabbies away!

DAY 124

Then he said unto them, Go your way, eat the fat, and drink the sweet, and send portions unto them for whom nothing is prepared: for this day is holy unto our LORD: neither be ye sorry; for the joy of the LORD is your strength.   NEHEMIAH 8:10

Patrick always hated programs on starving people around the world. The minute they would come on, he would turn off the television. What business was it of his if people halfway around the world were starving? He had all he needed, and he worked hard for it. So what if he was overweight? He earned that right because he was born in America!

The Bible teaches us that God gives us an abundance for just one reason: so that we will share it with those in need. If we take the bounty God offers and are selfish or gluttonous with it, then we are saying to God that we won't live as His children. We should take only what we need and share the rest, for that is the way of God.

TODAY'S THOUGHT: I have more than I need, and I don't really need much of what I want.

Day 125

But the salvation of the righteous is of the LORD: he is their strength in the time of trouble.   PSALM 37:39

Bob had a terrible dream. Food kept coming at him from every direction. Wherever it touched him, it stuck to him. Before long he couldn't move. He had trouble breathing. He had trouble seeing. He was hot and slimy. He kept trying to reach out for help, but no help came. He was buried under a mountain of food. As he lay awake thinking of the dream, he realized that it wasn't far from the truth. He was buried by a mountain of food become flesh. He did have trouble breathing and moving. It wasn't worth it. Silently, he reached out for help in a meek and humble prayer. God, the source of salvation, reached back.

TODAY'S THOUGHT: God, save me from an appetite seldom satisfied!

Day 126

Do all things without murmurings and disputings: That ye may be blameless and harmless, the sons of God, without rebuke, in the midst of a crooked and perverse nation, among whom ye shine as lights in the world.   PHILIPPIANS 2:14–15

Peggy kept looking at her daughter's trick-or-treat bag. Her daughter had made a grand haul of chocolates and sugary candies. It was all Peggy could do to keep her hands off it. A little devil inside kept telling her that her daughter wouldn't miss a few pieces. Peggy wanted to dive in so badly it hurt. She walked over to the bag and looked in. On its own, her hand moved toward the sweets. She was about to grab a handful when a still small voice stopped her. What had she been trying to teach her daughter about honesty and respecting things that weren't hers? Now she was attempting to pilfer her daughter's trick-or-treat bag because she wanted candy. When would she ever learn some strength and self-restraint?

TODAY'S THOUGHT: I will avoid things that make me less of a person but more of a body!

Day 127

For God is not unrighteous to forget your work and labour of love, which ye have shewed toward his name, in that ye have ministered to the saints, and do minister. HEBREWS 6:10

What a great reward! Robin had never looked so good. All her months of dieting paid off royally. It was beautiful to see the expressions on people's faces when they saw her. She couldn't wait to go out to show herself off. God had certainly blessed her through the rough time of dieting. There were days when she decided it just wasn't worth it. Now, she could hardly believe she ever had doubts. Looking in the mirror, she even surprised herself. She never thought she'd look this good.

When we dedicate ourselves to doing things that are right and good to do, God is sure to bless us and reward us for our labors.

TODAY'S THOUGHT: Improvement comes with practice. I can even get good at dieting!

Day 128

My brethren, count it all joy when ye fall into divers temptations. JAMES 1:2

Renee really felt good whenever she had the strength to say no to food that was offered to her. Each time she could refuse eating, it made her feel she'd won a moral victory. Mentally, she kept score. It became a game to see how often she could hold out between defeats. In a strange way, it made her diet enjoyable. She felt she was really accomplishing something that was important. By the end of about four months, Renee was able to defeat just about every temptation that came along. She felt God's pleasure as she grew more able to decline treats. That joy made her diet fly by.

TODAY'S THOUGHT: Diets can be fun, especially when they're done!

DAY 129

He that goeth forth and weepeth, bearing precious seed, shall doubt-less come again with rejoicing, bringing his sheaves with him.

PSALM 126:6

The groaning was over. The long nights of hunger lay behind. For some strange reason, the diet was getting easier. Finally, Diane's body had gotten the message that snacks and heavy meals were no more. The cravings and cryings of her stomach subsided. It had been a tough war, but Diane felt she had scored a victory at long last. All the weeping was behind, and she felt a wonderful joy. She knew that plenty of tough times lay ahead, but she also knew she could handle them. With God's help, she would make it. The hardest part was behind her.

TODAY'S THOUGHT: When I take it one day at a time, the days fall away as fast as the pounds!

DAY 130

Likewise, I say unto you, there is joy in the presence of the angels of God over one sinner that repenteth.

LUKE 15:10

Paul fumbled with his keys outside his apartment. When he tried the lock, the door swung inward. Cautiously, he entered. As he switched on the light, a dozen of his friends and neighbors jumped out, shouting, "Surprise!" They had come out to offer a congratulations party for the sixty pounds Paul had been able to lose. It was such a wonderful moment. Paul had felt joyful about what he had done for some time, but it was something special to have friends celebrate with him. God had blessed Paul so much. Not only had He helped him when he dieted, but He gave him such good friends.

TODAY'S THOUGHT: To gain means starvation; to lose, jubilation!

Day 131

Blessed are ye, when men shall revile you, and persecute you, and shall say all manner of evil against you falsely, for my sake.

MATTHEW 5:11

Ken could hardly wait to get back to school. Pete had ridden him about his weight the entire year before. When Ken had vowed to lose weight over the summer, Pete had laughed at him. "Fat boy, you can't keep away from food. You'll be back, big as a beach ball. Don't kid yourself!"

Ken could hardly wait to make Pete eat those words. He had spent the entire summer as a Christian youth counselor at camp. The people there were so supportive of what he was trying to do. They had made it possible. Not only had they helped him lose weight, but they helped him show Pete just how wrong he could be!

TODAY'S THOUGHT: I'm going to prove that there's more to me than my weight!

Day 132

And Jesus stood still, and commanded him to be called. And they call the blind man, saying unto him, Be of good comfort, rise; he calleth thee. And he, casting away his garment, rose, and came to Jesus.

MARK 10:49–50

Kate was so thankful. God had truly blessed her. She had been on the verge of collapse, and the doctor told her that her weight had to go. Reluctantly, she had started to diet, not expecting any great results. She prayed for God to help her, because she felt so weak. When the doctor gave her a clean bill of health, she closed her eyes and prayed.

God is God of the impossible. When we say "can't," He says "can." Faith is believing that God can, and will, help us when we are in need. God cares for His children, and for that we should be eternally grateful.

TODAY'S THOUGHT: I'd rather be grateful than have another plateful!

Day 133

But my God shall supply all your need according to his riches in glory by Christ Jesus.   PHILIPPIANS 4:19

It really wasn't fair that so many thin people couldn't understand what it meant to be fat. Patty got mad when thin friends chastised her for not sticking to her diet better. What did they know? Patty was always so thankful to God for what weight she'd been able to lose already that she could never understand why her friends put her down. Didn't they know what she had to sacrifice?

Whenever Patty got mad at her friends, she asked God to help calm her down. His peace filled her heart, and she was able to relax. God had done so much for her while she dieted. Too bad her friends couldn't see it.

TODAY'S THOUGHT: God is with me when it feels like the world is against me!

Day 134

For what thanks can we render to God again for you, for all the joy wherewith we joy for your sakes before our God? 1 THESSALONIANS 3:9

Gail wished she could do more for Mrs. Cooper. One night Mrs. Cooper had passed by her apartment and heard Gail crying. She stopped to see if there was anything she could do to help. Gail told her about her diet and how hard it was. Mrs. Cooper had been very sympathetic, and had spent many hours with her since. She helped take Gail's mind off food. Gail really felt strongly that she wouldn't have made it through the diet without Mrs. Cooper. We have someone who will listen to us when things get to be too much for us. That someone is God, and we can be thankful that He is ever with us, ready to listen to the concerns of our hearts.

TODAY'S THOUGHT: Let your praises to God be louder than the grumblings of your stomach!

DAY 135

Naked came I out of my mother's womb, and naked shall I return thither: the LORD gave, and the LORD hath taken away; blessed be the name of the LORD.   JOB 1:21

Stella was extremely frustrated. She had worked so hard to lose weight. She had done a great job, but now it was even harder to keep it off. She felt she was doing a good job of eating the right foods in small quantities, but when she'd step on the scales, she would find her weight creeping up. She always thought that once she got her weight down, everything would be easy. Boy, was that false! Weight-watching was a full-time job! Stella used to pray for God to keep her in line, but now the prayers were needed all the time. It just went to prove that nothing could be taken for granted. Good things don't come easy, but they're still worth having.

TODAY'S THOUGHT: Lord, give me strength, but take my weight problem!

DAY 136

And he answered and said unto them, I tell you that, if these should hold their peace, the stones would immediately cry out.   LUKE 19:40

Preston could hardly contain his excitement as the plane approached its landing. He hadn't seen his sister in over a year. At their last meeting he had weighed about 260 pounds. Now, he was a trim 180. He couldn't wait to see her face. He never remembered being so eager to see anyone before in his life. It was important to him to please his family, and he knew nothing would please his sister more than to see him looking so good.

God gives us such experiences to make our sacrifices worthwhile. We can be thankful that God motivates us in such loving ways. With His blessed help, we can't keep from succeeding.

TODAY'S THOUGHT: I want others to see me like they've never seen me before!

Day 137

Again, the kingdom of heaven is like unto treasure hid in a field; the which when a man hath found, he hideth, and for joy thereof goeth and selleth all that he hath, and buyeth that field. MATTHEW 13:44

Kris would give anything to be thin again. She was willing to diet; she was willing to exercise; she was willing to try anything. Following a number of traumatic experiences in her life, she had let herself go, but now she regretted it with all her heart. Earnestly she began to pray to God. Within a few weeks, her dieting was beginning to pay off. Delighted with the results, she doubled her efforts with her doctor's permission and devoted herself to her diet—body, mind, and soul. For the first time in years, she found herself happy and content. The joy she found was a blessed gift from God.

TODAY'S THOUGHT: I'm looking for little victories to keep me dieting!

Day 138

I thank my God, making mention of thee always in my prayers. . . . That the communication of thy faith may become effectual by the acknowledging of every good thing which is in you in Christ Jesus. PHILEMON 4, 6

Thomas was a great help with members of the group. He had lost so much weight, on more than one occasion, so he knew what it was like to triumph as well as to fall back into failure. He had rallied, though, and beaten his weight problem again. He was living proof that it could be done and that it wasn't hopeless when temptation got the better of a person. He shared his story with many people, and he helped them through some hard struggles. He was a faithful man, and his faith shone through. God had called Thomas to a very special ministry, and he answered that call in a very special way.

TODAY'S THOUGHT: I may fall back time and again, but I'm heading in the right direction!

Day 139

Whom having not seen, ye love; in whom, though now ye see him not, yet believing, ye rejoice with joy unspeakable and full of glory: Receiving the end of your faith, even the salvation of your souls.

1 Peter 1:8–9

Stephanie always had a picture in the back of her mind of what she would look like. She used to dream of how she would look once she lost weight. It was hard to imagine, but she did it anyway. That dream gave her motivation. Though she didn't really know what she'd look like, her imagination kept her on the right path.

Faith means acting on what we believe, even when we can't actually see the object of our faith. Faith in God teaches us how to put faith in action. When we are motivated by what we do not yet see, we find strength and joy in the living of our lives.

Today's thought: In my mind I see a whole new me!

Day 140

Looking unto Jesus the author and finisher of our faith; who for the joy that was set before him endured the cross, despising the shame, and is set down at the right hand of the throne of God.   Hebrews 12:2

Mary took comfort from the Gospels. Whenever she felt sorry for herself, she looked at the Bible. She couldn't believe all that Jesus had done and suffered. He had so much, and He emptied Himself to give to others. In the end, He received eternal glory. What a wonderful lesson. Dieting is a temporary and comparatively minor sacrifice, compared with Christ's sacrifice. And yet, as Christ triumphed over His situation, so shall we triumph over ours. Christ is our example in all things. The author and finisher of our faith has shown us the way to victory, and we share in His joy when we triumph in our own lives.

Today's thought: What I suffer today is worth the victory tomorrow!

DAY 141

*For he that is mighty hath done to me great things; and holy is his
name.* LUKE 1:49

Al sat in his chair, looking around the living room at all the people he
loved so much. Six months ago, he had almost died of a heart attack.
Today he was forty pounds trimmer and a whole lot healthier. He had
so much to be thankful for. God had been so good to him. He never
realized how much life meant to him until he almost lost it. Now he
found it wasn't that hard to watch his diet and his blood pressure. It
was worth it. God had done great things for Al. The least he could do
was take good care of himself. After all, he had a great family that he
planned to enjoy into his old, old age.

TODAY'S THOUGHT: Life is a gift from God that I have no right to
abuse!

DAY 142

*Praise ye the LORD. Praise the LORD, O my soul. . . . The LORD openeth
the eyes of the blind: the LORD raiseth them that are bowed down: the
LORD loveth the righteous.* PSALM 146:1, 8

Dick couldn't believe everyone was against him. First, his wife started
making comments about his weight. Next, it was his doctor. Now, his
friends at the office. He looked the same as he always had. Why was
everyone picking on him all of the sudden? Maybe he had gained a little, but that was just normal spread for a middle-aged man. He'd never
worried about weight before, and he sure wasn't planning to start wor-
rying now.

Sometimes we are too blind to see when we need to lose weight.
Pride gets in the way, and we aren't honest with ourselves. Ask God to
help keep ego out of the way, and He will open your eyes to see what
needs to be done.

TODAY'S THOUGHT: When it comes to weight, I won't kid myself!

Day 143

Sing unto the LORD; for he hath done excellent things: this is known in all the earth.   ISAIAH 12:5

Ann went out shopping for a whole new winter wardrobe. Every day of her diet, she had put money away for just this very day. She had set a goal for herself, and she promised to take herself shopping when she reached it. Now was that day, and she was overjoyed. For the first time in years, she wasn't embarrassed to go out for new things. She could walk into normal stores and pull things off the rack to wear. She could find new fashions and not worry about whether they came in her size. The whole world looked brighter. God had been so good to her, and she was thankful. Now she was going to be good to herself!

TODAY'S THOUGHT: I'm going to treat myself to a new me!

Day 144

And immediately he received his sight, and followed him, glorifying God: and all the people, when they saw it, gave praise unto God.
                                                                          LUKE 18:43

Scott knew his brother Dave couldn't have lost weight on his own. Dave had never been able to say no to food in all his life. When Scott asked Dave who helped him, Dave had just smiled and pointed up into the sky. Scott couldn't believe it. Dave was trying to tell him that God had made the transformation happen? Well, if that was true it would make a believer out of him. Scott had never been much of a Christian before, but if God could do that much for Dave, then He was someone worth believing in. The miracles of God truly are a wonder to behold.

TODAY'S THOUGHT: I will glorify God by losing weight for Him and for me!

Day 145

Jesus said unto her, I am the resurrection, and the life: he that believeth in me, though he were dead, yet shall he live.

JOHN 11:25

Ralph might as well have been dead. He never went out. He had few friends. He never felt like trying to do anything. He ate and drank and slept and went to work. What a life, if you could call it living. One day he couldn't bring himself to look at his own face in the mirror. Tearfully, he picked up the Bible his dead wife had given him some years before. As he read, he realized how he was throwing his life away. He was somebody important, if for no other reason than that God had made him. With a prayer of thanksgiving on his lips, Ralph decided to make a new start, and God's hand was upon him from that day forward.

TODAY'S THOUGHT: I want to live the life God wants me to live!

Day 146

Rejoice evermore.   1 THESSALONIANS 5:16

Fran remembered a time not long ago when she had nothing to smile about. She used to watch other women walk along, and bitter jealousy tore her up inside. She would fly into fits of rage and crying. She hated the way she looked, and she hated other women for looking so good. Her disposition was lousy, and her heart was broken. One Sunday she went to church, and while sitting there, she realized she was at peace. She closed her eyes and prayed, and she felt a voice tell her to change, to do something about her appearance. The impression was so strong that she went home immediately to plan a diet. From that time forward, she never wavered, and now she looked back in amazement. Seventy-five pounds lost, and joy filled the void they left.

TODAY'S THOUGHT: Happiness increases as my weight problem ceases!

Day 147

I called upon thy name, O LORD, out of the low dungeon. Thou hast heard my voice: hide not thine ear at my breathing, at my cry.
LAMENTATIONS 3:55–56

The dream was so real. Lew was standing in front of an old house where he could hear a witch cackling in the distance. He knew she was after him, but there was no place to hide. She flew around the corner of the house and touched his arm. At once he began to gain weight. Pound by pound mounted up, until he was a blob of flesh. He couldn't move, and the weight just kept coming. He became a prisoner within a mountainous body. He cried for help, and the clouds parted. A shaft of light came down, and the flesh began to melt. A gentle breeze blew, and Lew knew everything would be all right. When morning came, Lew vowed to lose the pounds he'd unnecessarily put on lately.

TODAY'S THOUGHT: From my fleshy prison, I have arisen!

Day 148

Praise ye the LORD: for it is good to sing praises unto our God; for it is pleasant; and praise is comely. . . . He healeth the broken in heart, and bindeth up their wounds.
PSALM 147:1, 3

It was more than a diet. For Gary, it was his sanity. He had been obsessed by his weight. He had lived the past three years in a deep and terrible depression. When he was at his lowest, God broke through to him. God turned Gary's life around. He finally began losing weight, and his state of mind improved dramatically. The light of God tore through his darkness with a beautiful healing warmth. Gary was healed of his physical affliction as well as the demon of depression that haunted him. God truly has the power to heal His children. No matter what the problem might be, take it to the Lord.

TODAY'S THOUGHT: My diet affects more than just my body; it affects my heart and mind, as well!

DAY 149

Again, the kingdom of heaven is like unto a merchant man, seeking goodly pearls: Who, when he had found one pearl of great price, went and sold all that he had, and bought it.   MATTHEW 13:45–46

A diet that worked! It wasn't anything fancy. It wasn't anything expensive. It didn't involve equipment or special treatments. In fact, it was a diet that anyone could do. Sally sat and talked with her pastor for about an hour, and he helped her see why she should diet for her own good, as well as for God. Her pastor has been a support for her ever since, and she has included God every step of the way. She feels stronger than ever before. It is like finding a treasure. She was so excited and so thankful. God has given her something that no one else can: a better figure *and* a deep, abiding joy.

TODAY'S THOUGHT: My weight will be lost, no matter the cost!

DAY 150

When they saw the star, they rejoiced with exceeding great joy.
MATTHEW 2:10

The star was the sign to the wise men that they were near their journey's end. They had followed the signs of the times, and they had been led toward Bethlehem. The star shone its light on their way, and they came to the Christ child.

As we diet, we can follow the light of Christ in our own lives. Christ shines His light on us to remind us of all we can be. His strength supports us along the way, and we come to possess His joy as we succeed in our quest. Nothing can keep the light of Christ from us, and, with Christ's help, nothing can keep us from losing weight.

TODAY'S THOUGHT: If God can lead travelers to the east to find Jesus, then He can lead me to a slimmer, trimmer me!

Day 151

And God saw their works, that they turned from their evil way; and God repented of the evil, that he had said that he would do unto them; and he did it not.
                                                        JONAH 3:10

Kent was devastated. The police review board had said he would be relieved of active duty if he didn't take off twenty pounds. He was a good cop. How could a few pounds make that much difference? Being a policeman was the most important thing in his life. If losing weight was what was required, then that's what he would do; no two ways about it.

God wants us to do whatever it takes to take care of ourselves. When we do what is right, we escape the bad consequences that come along. Kent knew what he had to do, and he did it. We know what we need to do, and with God's help we, too, will succeed.

TODAY'S THOUGHT: It's always a good idea to do what is pleasing to God!

Day 152

Then sang Moses and the children of Israel this song unto the LORD, and spake, saying, I will sing unto the LORD, for he hath triumphed gloriously: the horse and his rider hath he thrown into the sea.
                                                        EXODUS 15:1

The children of Israel were pursued by a great army as they came to the Red Sea. The Lord opened their way for them, then closed it up behind them, washing away the fighting force of Egypt. Moses and his followers were delivered, and the power of God was proven once more.

When we are oppressed by obesity, we can also call upon the Savior of Israel for salvation. The God who led His people out of captivity in Egypt will also lead His children of today out of captivity to fat. How can we doubt the power of God? With His help, all things are possible, if we will only believe.

TODAY'S THOUGHT: I'm breaking free from a body of fat!

DAY 153

I say unto you, that likewise joy shall be in heaven over one sinner that repenteth, more than over ninety and nine just persons, which need no repentance.   LUKE 15:7

Les dreaded Thanksgiving. He loved his family and friends, and he liked the parades and the football, and he even appreciated the day off from work, but he knew there would be so much tempting food that he wasn't supposed to have. It made him sick to think of all the wonderful things he would have to say no to. He walked up the front sidewalk and rang the bell. He was met by a dozen people who immediately went into raves over how great he looked. He was the topic of conversation the entire day. It wasn't so bad, after all. With everyone complimenting him, he found he had more strength than ever to turn down fattening food.

TODAY'S THOUGHT: God will send strength through family and friends!

DAY 154

And God saw every thing that he had made, and, behold, it was very good. And the evening and the morning were the sixth day.
                                        GENESIS 1:31

One thing that makes dieting so hard is that what we have to give up is so good. We have found ways to make foods into so many wonderful concoctions. It would be a lot easier to give up certain foods if they were drab and boring. Yet, variety is a true gift from God. We are given special treats to enjoy, but not to overindulge in. Gluttony robs life of its special treats. When we have whatever we want whenever we want it, then nothing is special anymore. If we will practice discipline and self-restraint, then we can treat ourselves to rich, luscious foods without worry of what they will do to us. That way, we come to enjoy treats the way God meant us to enjoy them.

TODAY'S THOUGHT: When I indulge too much, I bulge too much!

Day 155

And ye now therefore have sorrow: but I will see you again, and your heart shall rejoice, and your joy no man taketh from you.

JOHN 16:22

It was very weird, but Linda sort of missed her diet. She had made some really good friends in her weight-loss group, and she had gotten used to the routine. If anyone would have told her a few months ago that she would miss dieting, she would have said they were crazy. What was there to miss? She had freedom to eat more of what she wanted to now, and she didn't have to be self-conscious. Linda really believed that God had given her new friends and experiences for a reason. She was so thankful that she had been able to lose weight the way she did, with the people she did. Maybe now she could go back and be a help to others.

TODAY'S THOUGHT: On days when I can't help myself, maybe I can help others!

Day 156

Let every thing that hath breath praise the LORD. Praise ye the LORD.

PSALM 150:6

The battle wasn't won yet, but Henry felt it was close. He looked better, felt better, and had a more positive attitude. Life was so much more fun, now that he was thinner. All the really hard times were behind him, and he felt his future was pretty bright. God had certainly been good to him. Every day, Henry took time out to thank God for all He had done. Henry didn't know what he'd done to deserve such great blessings, but he wasn't going to question it too much. With God's help, he had been able to do what he could never do before: lose weight!

TODAY'S THOUGHT: God's helping me be both lighter of body and lighter of spirit!

DAY 157

Nay, in all these things we are more than conquerors through him that loved us.
ROMANS 8:37

Everyone was impressed with Annette's confidence. One day she announced that she was going on a diet, and she did just that. Over the course of the next few months, people watched the wondrous transformation take place. She had set her mind toward losing weight, and nothing even slowed her down. Such strength of conviction was a great inspiration for her friends.

God loves it when we stand up for something and will not be swayed. Whether it be a matter of faith or just of personal conviction, we are being true to our Creator when we triumph. Victory comes to those who walk in confidence.

TODAY'S THOUGHT: Without a doubt, fatness is out!

DAY 158

I press toward the mark for the prize of the high calling of God in Christ Jesus.
PHILIPPIANS 3:14

When he was young, Luke always came in last. He was never more than an average student; he had never succeeded much in anything he had done. That all changed when he decided to lose weight. He realized that much of his problem was a lousy self-image. He knew he could succeed, even if no one else believed it. He would prove it to himself, if nothing else. His pastor had given a sermon called, "Be everything you can be," and Luke was going to give it a shot. God didn't create losers. With God's help, Luke knew he could win. Nothing would stop him now. At long last, Luke was on the road to victory.

TODAY'S THOUGHT: I will try to keep my sight on what I want to be soon!

Day 159

For whatsoever is born of God overcometh the world: and this is the victory that overcometh the world, even our faith.   1 JOHN 5:4

Sammy was tired of making excuses. He was tired of being dishonest with himself and his friends. He needed to lose weight, and he needed plenty of help to do it. He was considered a strong member of his church, but he didn't even have enough faith or conviction to take off a few pounds. He felt like a hypocrite. Surely, the God who had given him so much strength in other areas of his life could help him lose weight. Christ had conquered so very much. Sammy felt he ought to be able to conquer so very little. Prayerfully, he began a journey toward fitness, assured of the victory through his faith in Christ.

TODAY'S THOUGHT: A heart full of Christ is more important than a plate full of food!

Day 160

Let us draw near with a true heart in full assurance of faith, having our hearts sprinkled from an evil conscience, and our bodies washed with pure water.   HEBREWS 10:22

Betty liked having people around. When others watched her, she was more likely to behave herself and stay on her diet. She felt guilty if anyone caught her cheating. A little guilt was a good thing for someone trying to lose weight. When she was alone, she didn't feel nearly as guilty. If she was ever going to lose weight, she was going to have to make sure there were people around.

We ought to remember that no matter what we do, God is watching. He can help us on to victory if we will keep in mind that He is ever with us, to act as our conscience when we need Him to.

TODAY'S THOUGHT: I hope my conscience is stronger than my appetite!

DAY 161

Blessed is the man that endureth temptation: for when he is tried, he shall receive the crown of life, which the Lord hath promised to them that love him.   JAMES 1:12

Shelley was thrilled when she was named homecoming queen. It had been a dream of hers since childhood. When she knew she was in the running, she began to diet. Weight had always been a struggle for her. This time she had great motivation, and that made all the difference in the world. She prayed for God's help, and He gave her the determination she needed to diet—and to win the crown. The crown of the pageant was one thing, but Shelley knew God had given her much more than that. Through faith, she had received life everlasting and a share in the victory of Christ Jesus.

TODAY'S THOUGHT: My diet will end, but the lessons learned from it will last a lifetime!

DAY 162

For thou, LORD, hast made me glad through thy work: I will triumph in the works of thy hands.   PSALM 92:4

Brent never knew how happy he would be when he lost weight. All his life he had toyed with the idea, but the costs always seemed much greater than the benefits. It wasn't until the weight came off that he truly realized how great being thinner really was. He felt better; he looked better, and he enjoyed life in general so much more. He could do things he'd never dreamed of before. Even picking things up off the floor without panting and groaning gave him special pleasure. Brent couldn't thank God enough for helping him find a new life. It was great to be alive!

TODAY'S THOUGHT: God makes the joy greater than any amount of sacrifice!

Day 163

Then Job answered the LORD, and said, I know that thou canst do every thing, and that no thought can be withholden from thee.

JOB 42:1–2

Blessed assurance. Why do some people seem to have it while others don't? It stems from a very slight difference. Some people know God, and some just believe in Him. Knowing is belief beyond doubt. True confidence in the Lord comes to those who have moved beyond their doubts. When we defeat doubt, then we can enter into a whole new relationship with God and a whole new life. God is greater than any problem we have. If we want to lose weight and want God to help us, we need to know beyond a doubt that He will truly help us. Like Job, we need to confess regularly our belief that God can do everything.

TODAY'S THOUGHT: If God could create mountains, then He can remove a pound of flesh from me!

Day 164

The LORD thy God in the midst of thee is mighty; he will save, he will rejoice over thee with joy; he will rest in his love, he will joy over thee with singing.

ZEPHANIAH 3:17

Toni had a dream that she was entering a room where God was. She couldn't really see Him, but she knew He was there. For some reason, He was very happy with her. He was making her feel very good, and she could tell she had done something to please Him a lot. When she gathered up her nerve, Toni asked God what she had done to make Him so happy. "Lost weight," was the reply. When she awakened, she felt the greatest joy she had ever known. She had really wanted to lose weight for herself, but to think that God was pleased with what she had done made the victory twice as sweet.

TODAY'S THOUGHT: I will rejoice with God as the pounds come off!

DAY 165

And it shall come to pass, that whosoever shall call on the name of the Lord shall be saved.   ACTS 2:21

Barbara was so thankful. She had come so far, but lately the stress had been overwhelming. When she was under stress, she liked to eat. She was so afraid of blowing her diet that it just added to the stress. She was nervous and on edge all the time. One evening, while she had some time alone, she settled down to read her Bible and pray. It was one of the most peaceful experiences she had had in weeks. She felt renewed and strengthened by the experience—so much so that she made it a nightly routine. It got her through the stress, and it kept her on her diet. By God's grace she triumphed.

TODAY'S THOUGHT: I admit I need help, but it's good to know that God offers all the help I can handle!

DAY 166

For the kingdom of God is not meat and drink; but righteousness, and peace, and joy in the Holy Ghost.   ROMANS 14:17

Joan's doctor had told her to make a list of what was really important to her. Her husband and children headed the list. Her health was next, then her pets. She also wrote down her mother's ring and some furniture that her father had made when he was a young man. Her doctor asked her if she wanted to lose all that was on the list, and she told him "Of course not!" He told her that she had to lose weight or she wouldn't be around long to enjoy the things she truly loved. If those things were really more important to her than food, then she was going to have to prove it. She asked God for help and then set her mind toward losing weight.

TODAY'S THOUGHT: Compared to the truly important things in life, food is pretty pathetic!

Day 167

But he that doeth truth cometh to the light, that his deeds may be made manifest, that they are wrought in God. JOHN 3:21

Jack was so proud to show off his wife, Eileen, when they went home for the holidays. Over the summer and fall, she had lost sixty-five pounds. She looked great, and Jack was proud of her. She had worked so hard, and he felt she deserved some credit. It made Eileen feel good to know it meant so much to Jack. God had been good to them both. He had given them patience to deal with each other and had blessed them both with strength and encouragement. It was true that when a person worked to do what the Lord wanted her to do, He crowned her in victory and allowed her to bask in the limelight for awhile!

TODAY'S THOUGHT: I don't care if I come into the limelight, as long as I become light!

Day 168

Blessed are the pure in heart: for they shall see God.
MATTHEW 5:8

Denise wanted to do what was right. She was a good person, and it never occurred to her that her weight problem might be displeasing to God. Her friend tried to tell her that it didn't mean God didn't love her. What she meant was that God likes it best when we take the best care of ourselves possible, and that extra weight wasn't doing that. Denise pondered what her friend said to her for a long while, then resolved to try her best to lose weight. Apologetically, she prayed to God and asked Him to help her as she tried to set things right. The prayer of a person pure in heart and full of kindness speaks loudest into the ear of the Lord.

TODAY'S THOUGHT: I wish my heart could teach my mouth to say "no"!

DAY 169

*He that hath an ear, let him hear what the Spirit saith unto the churches;
To him that overcometh will I give to eat of the tree of life, which is in
the midst of the paradise of God.*   REVELATION 2:7

Beth and David made a deal that they would diet through the week but
treat themselves to a night out each week at one of their favorite restau-
rants. Restaurant night became the best night of the week. Both Beth
and David agreed that they had never enjoyed their food so much as
when they only splurged one time a week. They grew to appreciate
how good it really was. It helped to make even ordinary meals special
and delicious.

God has offered us special things to eat. He has created so much to
make our lives interesting and varied. We must enjoy these things dis-
creetly and unselfishly. If we will enjoy them within God's plan, then
He will reward us with fruit from the tree of life, which will be the finest
food we could ever want.

TODAY'S THOUGHT: God's food is eternal, and it isn't fattening!

DAY 170

*For ye have need of patience, that, after ye have done the will of God,
ye might receive the promise.*   HEBREWS 10:36

Paula woke up in pain. Her stomach was cramping, and she felt ill. It
must have been the diet pills. Her friend had told her they were safe, and
they'd help take off weight three times as fast as normal. Why had she
listened to her? She knew pills weren't the answer, but she wanted to
lose weight fast. She never had been very good at patience. Her mother
told her to pray for patience, but no, Paula thought she had a better idea.
The truth was, there was only one way she was going to lose weight, and
that was through perseverance and patience. Her mother was right. If
God would give her a second chance, maybe together they could make
it work.

TODAY'S THOUGHT: Nothing takes off weight faster than devotion
and commitment!

Day 171

For he that is mighty hath done to me great things; and holy is his name. LUKE 1:49

Carolyn felt good about herself. She was in her own apartment, working full-time at a job she loved, and she was looking better than ever before. God had been so good to her. She was afraid when she first set out on her own, but she knew He was looking after her. With God on her side, she felt she could accomplish anything. God had set her feet on a good road, and she was going to try her hardest to stick to it. She wanted everyone to know what God had done for her, and she planned to do nothing that would allow anyone to doubt. The power of God shone brightly through her life, and she was glad.

TODAY'S THOUGHT: I want my diet to be a sign of God's grace!

Day 172

Blessed be the Lord, who daily loadeth us with benefits, even the God of our salvation. Selah. PSALM 68:19

Doris stood at the window, watching the first heavy snow cover everything outside with a blanket of white. She sipped a cup of tea and reflected on the year quickly fleeting. So many good things had happened. Certainly there had been bad, too, but mostly it was good. She couldn't imagine why she was so blessed as to have so many things going her way. The Lord had looked kindly on her this year. She had never felt so healthy and good. The year had seen weight loss every month. She finally was beginning to look like she'd always dreamed she could. The Lord could take credit for that, too. There was no way Doris could have done so well if God hadn't strengthened her.

TODAY'S THOUGHT: I gladly receive all the benefits the Lord has to give, as long as they're not fattening!

DAY 173

Know ye not that they which run in a race run all, but one receiveth the prize? So run, that ye may obtain. 1 CORINTHIANS 9:24

Todd wasn't getting anywhere with his diet. It was on and off, at best. He just couldn't stick to it. He'd never been good at discipline and conditioning. How many times had he been kicked off high school teams for not practicing? He just didn't have the killer instinct. He didn't want to win badly enough.

We'll have difficulty losing weight if our heart isn't really in it. If we're going to run the race for weight loss, then we need to be serious about winning it. Pray that God will strengthen both your heart and body, so that when the race is finished, you'll receive the prize.

TODAY'S THOUGHT: Help me remember that I'm not just running away from fat, but that I'm running toward God's design of who I should be!

DAY 174

Herein is love, not that we loved God, but that he loved us, and sent his Son to be the propitiation for our sins. 1 JOHN 4:10

God has given all to make us happy. He has blessed us with a beautiful world, a wonderful life, and many opportunities for fulfillment and joy. He asks that we respect His gifts and endeavor to be the best people we can possibly be. To help us, He sent His only Son to come into this world as an example. We can know God's desire for us through His Son. Not only did His Son come as an example, but as a Savior, to allow us to be reconciled with our God. All that we have received is from God. This morning, make a gift of your life to God. Give Him the only thing that truly matters: *You!*

TODAY'S THOUGHT: If I can in any way be used, help me bring about peace on earth and goodwill to all God's children!

Day 175

For our light affliction, which is but for a moment, worketh for us a far more exceeding and eternal weight of glory.   2 CORINTHIANS 4:17

The army had been good for Stan. When he was younger, he was completely undisciplined. The army had taken care of that. He had to work his tail off to get into good shape, but it was worth it. The short period of affliction he suffered through helped him in so many other ways. The folks back home couldn't believe the change they saw while he was home for the holidays.

God disciplines His children on occasion because He knows the lasting lessons we need to learn. Diets help us grow in maturity and fitness for the kingdom of God.

TODAY'S THOUGHT: A gain in discipline means a loss in weight!

Day 176

He that hath an ear, let him hear what the Spirit saith unto the churches; To him that overcometh will I give to eat of the hidden manna, and will give him a white stone, and in the stone a new name written, which no man knoweth saving he that receiveth it.

REVELATION 2:17

Donna thanked God for giving her a whole new life. Losing the weight had only been part of it. Donna had fervently prayed for transformation, but she never bargained for all that God would do for her. Her attitude was transformed from one of doom to one of hope. Her appearance was transformed from one of dumpiness to one of beauty. Her emotional stability had been transformed from one of teetering on the brink to solid rock. She couldn't believe it, but she was a totally different person than she had been a year before. The God of miracles and life had certainly worked in Donna's life. He's available to work in ours, also.

TODAY'S THOUGHT: With God's help I will lose weight, lose hate, and lose my desire to denigrate!

Day 177

Who is he that overcometh the world, but he that believeth that Jesus is the Son of God?   1 John 5:5

Burt couldn't help but rub it in. Terry had claimed to have found the diet breakthrough of the century. He lost seven pounds. Greg got hold of some miracle pills, and he lost eleven pounds. Craig had mortgaged his house to buy a membership in a health club. He managed to lose fourteen pounds. Burt had simply told his friends he was going to lose weight on the Jesus plan. Whenever he got hungry between meals, he was going to go off and read the Gospels. They had all laughed long and hard at him, but he who laughs last, laughs best. Twenty-eight pounds had dropped because of the Jesus plan. There's nothing like it.

TODAY'S THOUGHT: God can do for me what nothing on earth can!

Day 178

Then the devil leaveth him, and, behold, angels came and ministered unto him.   Matthew 4:11

Victory! Steve felt he'd really run the good race. No matter how great the temptations had gotten lately, he had been able to withstand them. Christ was pulling him through the roughest times yet. Each time he beat back the temptations, he felt better than ever. It was as if God was rewarding him by making him feel so good. The pounds were coming off, and it was actually beginning to get easy. Steve never thought he'd come to say that. Steve was convinced. If God could make a diet tolerable, then God really could do anything!

TODAY'S THOUGHT: I will not take part in the devil's food!

Day 179

Whether therefore ye eat, or drink, or whatsoever ye do, do all to the glory of God.   1 CORINTHIANS 10:31

Leah remembered the question her pastor had asked, "What do you think God wants you to eat?" At first, it had seemed like a silly question, but the more Leah thought about it, the more she realized there really wasn't any food God didn't want to let her have. It was the quantities and frequency of consumption that Leah realized God would disapprove of. Moderation in everything was the rule she needed to follow. She felt so much better. Her diet didn't need to be a lot of heavy sacrifices. All she needed to do was develop some self-control, and with God's help, she would.

TODAY'S THOUGHT: Let my eating and drinking offend no one, especially God!

Day 180

Go thy way, eat thy bread with joy, and drink thy wine with a merry heart; for God now accepteth thy works.   ECCLESIASTES 9:7

There will come a day when the diet is truly over. We must endure until that day with a strong spirit and an earnest desire to please the Lord. We have been blessed with much, and in some cases, too much. God has been good to give, and He will be equally good to help take away. Remember the Lord every step of your diet. Call upon Him for strength, for comfort, for hope, and for courage. He will hear you, and He will be sure to answer you. In time, you will come to that day, not too distant, when you can eat your bread with joy and without guilt, drink and make merry, and stand confident and proud that you have indeed glorified your Lord.

TODAY'S THOUGHT: I will be a conqueror, through the mighty love of God.

*May the peace of God
abide with you always,
the love of Christ protect you
from the storms of life,
and the power of the Holy Spirit
strengthen you all the days
of your life.
Amen.*

FOR
ADDITIONAL
INSPIRATION

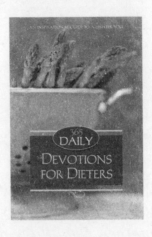

365 Daily Devotions for Dieters is a must-have daily devotional that gives the encouragement necessary for successful dieting. With monthly topics like temptation, patience, and perseverance, dieters will find uplifting scripture, devotions, and thoughts for every day of the year.

ISBN 978-1-59789-690-0

384 pages, $7.97

Available wherever books are sold.